PRAISE FOR

The Autoimmune
Wellness Handbook

"Packed to the gills with applicable solutions, *The Autoimmune Wellness Handbook* is my new favorite resource for today's #1 emerging health challenge. If you or a loved one suffers from autoimmunity and aren't sure where to begin—START HERE."

—Russ Crandall, *New York Times*-bestselling author of *Paleo Takeout*
    and *The Ancestral Table*

"It is normal to meet an autoimmune diagnosis with a tremendous sense of confusion, loss, and betrayal, and the information overwhelm can leave the initiate tumbling in its wake. This is where Mickey and Angie's book comes in. *The Autoimmune Wellness Handbook* is an elegant and encouraging guide that not only succinctly reviews the nuts and bolts of autoimmune disease management but also leads you through an often tumultuous inner journey with loving wisdom. In its own unforgiving way, autoimmune diseases force us to honor human design, not society's (often shaming) version. The autoimmune patient must learn to rest, self-advocate, love and be loved, self-nourish, move appropriately, release toxic people and situations, and lift the veil on buried shadows. Like all of life's best rewards, autoimmune management is hard-won. But, as this handbook shows you, the autoimmune journey can also be an enriching path to a more authentic you."

—Datis Kharrazian, author of *Why Do I Still Have Thyroid Symptoms?*
    and *Why Isn't My Brain Working?*

"*The Autoimmune Wellness Handbook* offers a powerful—yet safe and drug-free— approach to the millions of people now suffering from autoimmune diseases. Mickey and Angie recognize that diet is the the cornerstone of managing autoimmune disease, but they also know that stress management, sleep, pleasure, and living a rich and rewarding life can be just as important. I can't recommend this book highly enough."

—Chris Kresser, MS, LAc, *New York Times* bestselling author of
    Your Personal Paleo Code

"When I think of a *guide* book, I think of a fishing guide, a travel guide, a study guide...a book that shows me the way to do something. As the title lists, *The Autoimmune Wellness Handbook* is a do-it-yourself guide to living well with chronic illness. I would take exception to this title. As I read this book, I found it to be not only a masterfully written guide but much more. It's more than a journal and personal inside-scoop of two people who have found the path back to health. This book is in a category of its own.

"It's not just a guide; it's more of a health missal-a book containing all instructions and texts necessary for the celebration of life when addressing a chronic illness.

"In my opinion, they've found the right path back to health that has the potential to help hundreds of thousands. Read this book and you will understand what it takes to put a disease into remission and keep it there. Thank you to Mickey Trescott and Angie Alt for this inspiring road map to living well in this toxic world we have inherited."

—Tom O'Bryan, DC, CCN, DACBN

"An autoimmune diagnosis can knock our world on its side, leaving us hurting, scared, and confused. This book is a guide through that darkness, back into the light again. Mickey and Angie have walked this path themselves and helped thousands of others do the same. They've taken all of their personal experience and professional knowledge and created a thorough workbook for creating a healthy, vital, joyful life again. Our story doesn't have to stop with our diagnosis. In many ways, it's a new beginning."

—Eileen Laird, author of *The Simple Guide to the Paleo Autoimmune Protocol*

"Mickey and Angie have created something wonderful: an unapologetically empowering guide to everything autoimmune that lets you know you're not alone. *The Autoimmune Wellness Handbook* is a true companion, friend, and advocate for anyone wanting to live vibrantly in the face of autoimmune disease."

—Rachael Bryant, author of *Nourish: The Paleo Healing Cookbook*

the Autoimmune Wellness

HANDBOOK

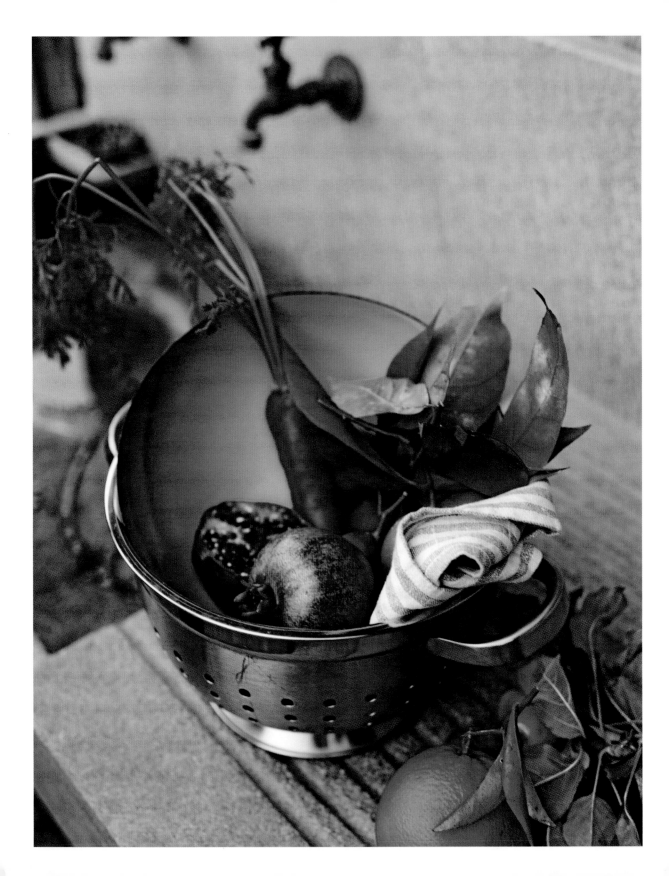

the Autoimmune Wellness
HANDBOOK

A DIY GUIDE TO LIVING WELL
WITH CHRONIC ILLNESS

MICKEY TRESCOTT, NTP, AND **ANGIE ALT**, NTC, CHC
FOUNDERS OF AUTOIMMUNE-PALEO.COM

RODALE

RODALE
wellness

Live happy. Be healthy. Get inspired.

Sign up today to get exclusive access to our authors, exclusive bonuses,
and the most authoritative, useful, and cutting-edge information on health,
wellness, fitness, and living your life to the fullest.

Visit us online at RodaleWellness.com

Join us at RodaleWellness.com/Join

Rodale books may be purchased for business or promotional use or for special sales.
For information, please write to:
Special Markets Department, Rodale Inc., 733 Third Avenue, New York, NY 10017

Printed in China

Rodale Inc. makes every effort to use acid-free ♾, recycled paper ♻.

Photographs by Charlotte Dupont

Book design by Joanna Williams

Library of Congress Cataloging-in-Publication Data is on file with the publisher.

ISBN 978-1-62336-729-9 paperback

Distributed to the trade by Macmillan

6 8 10 9 7 5 paperback

 RODALE

Follow us @RodaleBooks on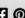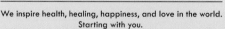

We inspire health, healing, happiness, and love in the world.
Starting with you.

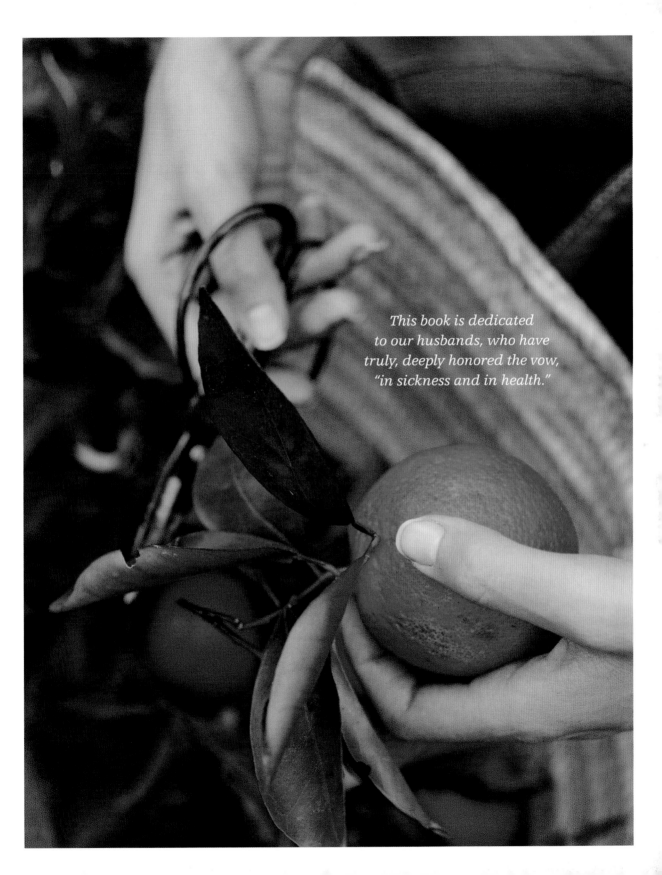

*This book is dedicated
to our husbands, who have
truly, deeply honored the vow,
"in sickness and in health."*

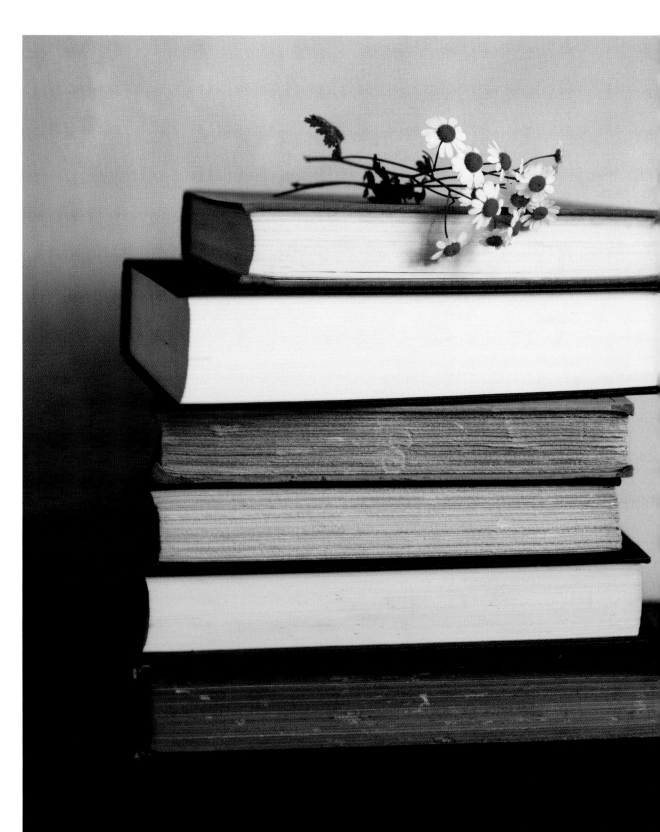

Contents

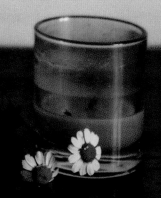

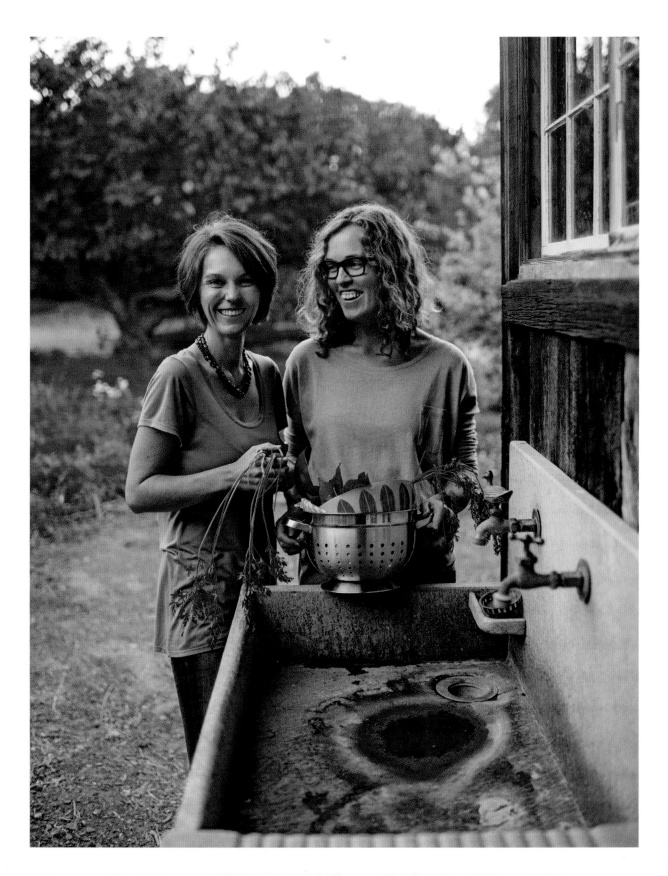

Introduction

MOST PEOPLE'S AUTOIMMUNE STORIES START THE same way, with a trickle of strange, seemingly disconnected symptoms—things like increasing fatigue, joint pain, or more frequent headaches. In time, the trickle becomes a steady stream that exists as background noise in our daily lives. After repeated and desperate attempts to explain the symptoms to dismissive doctors, most of us resolve to silently suffer. Later, the steady stream becomes an undeniable flood, and with it comes the sensation that you are drowning in an unnamed illness. At this late stage, doctors may finally have a diagnosis, but follow-up, if it is even offered, consists of limited treatment options with disabling side effects. Feeling hopeless and demoralized is standard for those with autoimmune disease, and it is probably why you have this book in your hands right now. If you follow the conventional approach, living *well* with autoimmune disease is rarely achievable.

We are proposing an alternate way of thinking about autoimmune disease and health care in general: patient-centered, guided by self-discovery, informed, and proactive. This is a stark contrast to the typical experience that leaves patients feeling fearful, anxious, and demeaned. In order to live well with chronic illness, you need to become a *new* kind of patient, one who is savvy enough to know that a whole-body approach is necessary. You can redefine the process by empowering and informing yourself, combining the best of medical care with dietary and lifestyle modifications. Despite the current standard of care, *it is possible to live vibrantly in the face of autoimmune disease*!

With five autoimmune diseases between us, this is exactly the process we, the authors, have used in our own lives with astounding results. Through years of experience, we have refined the tools and resources we used and aim to share that knowledge with you, someone who is ready to take personal responsibility for your health and wellness. But where do you start?

The Autoimmune Wellness Handbook encompasses seven key steps on the autoimmune path: *inform, collaborate, nourish, rest, breathe, move,* and *connect*. These verbs elegantly describe the simple actions that you can take to achieve wellness, despite autoimmune disease. This book is about demystifying and breaking down what can be a very complex, overwhelming, and isolating process, and replacing it with one that is clear and liberating. Through the use of practical tools, resources, and self-assessments, you can begin your own journey of recovery by setting yourself up for success.

First, you'll *inform* yourself by determining where on the spectrum of illness you lie. You'll recognize the importance of diagnosis and educate yourself about your autoimmune disease, including testing, treatment options, and prognosis. You'll then learn how to *collaborate*, educating yourself on the difference between natural and conventional approaches, as well as how to assemble your health-care team. You'll go on to prioritize each step of your journey, including how to approach your own medical situation, and identify when medications, treatments, and surgery are necessary.

Once you complete the steps of informing and collaborating, you move on to a central part of the process, in which you *nourish* your body in order to recover from autoimmune disease. Here, you'll discover the relationship of the gut to autoimmune disease, why there is no one-size-fits-all approach to diet, and why an elimination and reintroduction protocol, in the form of the Autoimmune Protocol, is the best place to start to get to the root of food-driven symptoms. We'll show you how to transition your diet, how to explore food reintroductions, and why balance matters when approaching what's on your plate.

Continuing your journey, you'll put the pieces together and grasp how to truly *rest* and *breathe*. Details will be uncovered about why sleep and stress management matter. In the next section, you'll learn how to optimally *move*, with assessments designed to pinpoint if you are under- or overdoing activities and how to come up with a plan that supports your goals. To tie it up, you'll *connect*, both with others and the natural world. This section of the healing journey is often overlooked, but you will learn why it is a crucial part of recovery.

As much as we'd like to give you all the answers, what we have found is that there is no standard formula. Self-discovery and individuality are the missing ingredients in most gurus' schemes. Instead, we are presenting a handbook for uncovering solutions that will be specific to *your* unique healing journey. As Bruce Lee famously said, "Absorb what is useful, discard what is useless, add what is essentially your own." We are advocating a way to take the best of a broken system and combine it with self-empowerment. The path we are suggesting is challenging, but also rewarding; by following it, you will find a true sense of balance and allow the joy of discovery to transform your life.

The Autoimmune Wellness Handbook combines knowledge with action and pioneers a new era in how autoimmune diseases are viewed and treated. You can join us by taking ownership of this phase of your life. From participating in your medical care to deciding what is on your plate, empowerment can guide you to make the choices that spark true health. The tide is already turning, the shift is under way—what you stand to gain from this book is vibrant health that will outlast the hype!

WHY WE WROTE THIS BOOK

Living well with autoimmune disease can seem daunting or downright impossible, but our healing stories prove otherwise. Like you, we've also been at the base of this mountain gazing at the pinnacle and wondering if there is a route to the top. While we coach people through recovery using diet and lifestyle in our professional lives, it is actually our personal journeys as patients that breathe heart into this book. We've been in your shoes with autoimmune disease, and first, we'd like to share how our experiences inspired this unique approach.

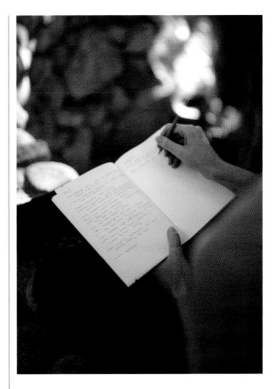

Our own paths to diagnosis were long and complex. After experiencing troubling symptoms, Mickey worked with five different doctors (all of whom told her everything was "normal") before getting her primary diagnosis of Hashimoto's thyroiditis. Angie developed symptoms 11 years before her primary diagnosis of celiac disease. It took doctors on three continents and eventually some of the most advanced medical centers in the United States to get an answer. Sadly, these runarounds are often the norm for autoimmune patients.

Even though getting a diagnosis helped us understand what was going on in our bodies, it didn't change the severity of the symptoms we were experiencing. Mickey was undergoing a major health crisis and was no longer able to work. She was dealing with unrelenting fatigue, brain fog, dizziness, vertigo, insomnia, neuropathy, and joint pain. Angie was so ill that her family had to relocate from their dream position overseas. She, too, was unable to work and dropped out of school because she was experiencing symptoms like numbness all over her body, slurred speech, anxiety, panic attacks, muscle wasting, and extreme bone pain. These symptoms were powerful motivators for us both to seek deeper answers. We came to the realization, on our own, that we had to rely on ourselves to come up with a more comprehensive recovery plan.

At the time, we both felt isolated, defeated, and overwhelmed looking at the road before us. Through searching online, we discovered the Autoimmune Protocol, and in our desperation, became two of the first people to try it. Once we started making dietary changes, it was clear almost immediately that this was going to be a powerful component to healing, and we both started blogging about those early "wins." Later, we discovered that recovery was not only about food but also it needed to involve collaboration with our health-care teams and adopting a healing lifestyle. Through finding the right combination of conventional, natural, and DIY approaches,

implemented gradually over the course of 4 years, both of us have completely regained our health and happiness and are able to live full, vibrant lives.

We've had a chance to look back on all the things we tried: what worked, what didn't, and what we wished we had known sooner. Now, we get out of bed every morning with one thing on our minds, "How am I going to make this easier for the next person?" The way we view and treat autoimmune disease in this country and all around the world is undergoing a revolution, and you can be part of it! We wrote this book to put the innovative tools we use in your hands and to convince you that living well with autoimmune disease is more than a possibility—it can be your future, too.

OUR EXPERIENCE

If we chronicled all of the details of our journeys, it would be a whole separate book! Instead, we've decided to give you glimpses into our experiences through these boxes in relevant areas throughout the book. It is our hope that through honest, open sharing, we can help you feel less alone in this process, provide a realistic lens for viewing autoimmune wellness, and help you recognize that this approach was not always simple or easy for us.

The Manifesto

You're about to get into the details and begin applying the principles we lay out in this book. Before we go there, perspective on the larger health movement you are about to join can provide a welcome sense of community and motivation before you embark.

1. **TRUST YOUR INTUITION.** You don't need a guru to navigate this process successfully.

2. **EMBRACE THE TEMPLATE.** The Autoimmune Protocol is not one-size-fits-all; it's a template that promotes individuality and self-discovery.

3. **INFORMATION IS POWER.** Learn enough to be an informed and proactive advocate for your health.

4. **START SIMPLE.** Begin with the foundations of diet, sleep, stress management, movement, and relationships before delving deeper.

5. **TAKE IT SLOW.** Don't be afraid to make changes in phases—it was the tortoise and not the hare that won the race!

6. **FOOD IS YOUR FRIEND.** It provides nourishment to every single cell in your body!

7. **SET YOURSELF UP FOR SUCCESS.** Planning and preparation are the keys.

8. **BE A NUTRIENT SEEKER.** Don't ignore the foods that accelerate healing and restore health.

9. **FOOD OVER SUPPLEMENTS.** Nutrients are often synergistic and more potent in nature's packaging.

10. **DON'T DIET "HARDER."** Resist the temptation to further restrict instead of troubleshoot.

11. **SEEK HELP.** When necessary, thoughtfully add practitioners to your team who don't undermine your authority.

12. **TEST, DON'T GUESS.** Always use testing to reveal root issues, if progress is not as expected.

13. **BE SKEPTICAL.** "Magic bullets" that only the elite can afford are not the solution to our health-care crisis.

14. **STRIVE FOR BALANCE.** Restoring your health is a worthy pursuit, but it is not a religion.

15. **SUPPORT IS CRUCIAL.** If your networks aren't strong enough, explore ways to add to your human connections.

16. **REFRAME THE NEGATIVES.** Find areas where your life has been expanded by your experience with illness.

17. **PRACTICE GRATITUDE.** Give thought energy to what is good in your life.

18. **KEEP YOUR EYES ON YOUR OWN JOURNEY.** The path to wellness is unique for all of us. Resist the urge to compare.

19. **HEALTH BEFORE IMAGE.** Value wellness above numbers on a scale or reflections in a mirror.

20. **VIBRANT HEALTH IS A LIFELONG JOURNEY.** Nobody ever regrets investing in his or her own wellness. Enjoy the process of restoring your health!

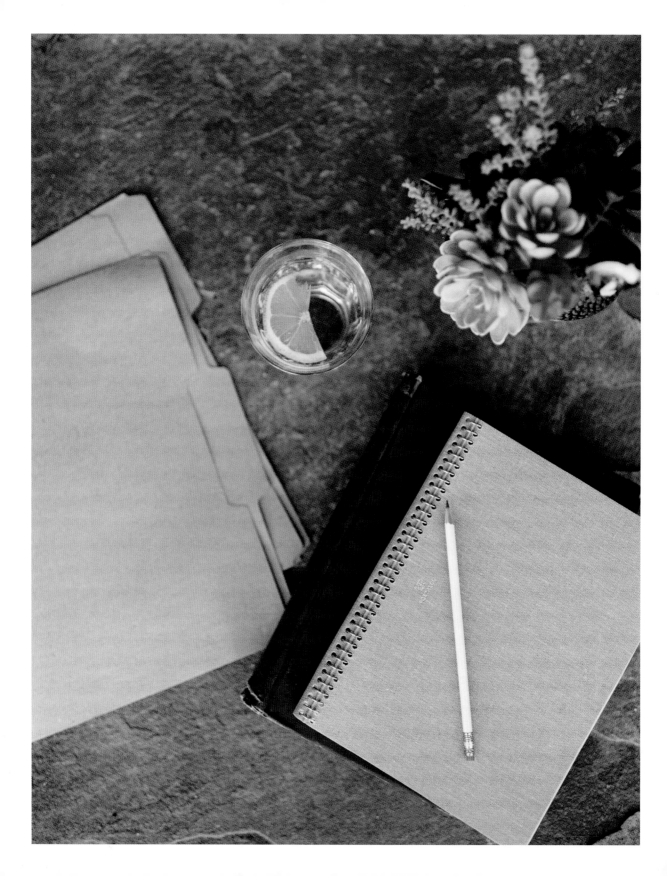

CHAPTER 1

Inform

*"Nothing in life is to be feared, it is only to be understood." —*MARIE CURIE

THE FIRST STEP TO LIVING WELL with autoimmune disease is being informed about your illness. We have chosen this as the first step, because the burden of truly understanding lies with you. Although there is a lot of information to be gained in working with a skilled doctor, relying on him or her to also be your teacher detracts from your personal responsibility in healing. You may find learning the details about your disease to be unnerving, because knowing makes it hard to hide from your new reality. After the initial fear subsides, understanding inspires a level of courage you previously didn't have and empowers you to take control of your health and start on the path toward healing. In this chapter, we aim to give you an overview of what autoimmune disease is, how to get and cope with a diagnosis, the different treatments you might expect, and how to gather and store information.

WHAT IS AUTOIMMUNE DISEASE?

Simply put, autoimmune disease occurs when your immune system, which is designed to protect you from foreign invaders (pathogens like viruses and bacteria), starts attacking your own tissue. This is done through the creation of antibodies, which are ordinarily used to identify and destroy pathogens and help you recover from an illness. In the case of autoimmunity, however, these antibodies target your own healthy tissue, which leads to inflammation and destruction of your cells. This is like your own team playing against you— not fair!

The American Autoimmune Related Diseases Association (AARDA) estimates that more than 50 million Americans (roughly 1 in 6) suffer from autoimmune diseases, 75 percent of which are women. Medical science has identified more than 100 autoimmune diseases, with another 40 suspected to have an autoimmune component. Autoimmune disease is one of the most significant health-care issues facing our world today. According to the AARDA, in the United States alone, more than $100 billion is spent annually on the conventional treatment of this condition. Its incidence is on the rise, with some disease prevalence tripling in the last decade. It remains poorly understood, with no medical specialty to support it and a severe lack of research funding, as well as treatment options that only manage symptoms, but do not produce lasting wellness.

Autoimmune disease can involve any organ or system in your body, including joint, skin, digestive, hormonal, connective, nerve, and muscle tissues. If you have rheumatoid arthritis, your joints are affected; if you have Hashimoto's thyroiditis, it's your thyroid; and if it's multiple sclerosis, the myelin, the protective layer around your nerves, is destroyed. While it may seem that these conditions are vastly different, the common thread of an immune system gone haywire links them together. Often, autoimmune disease affects multiple organs or systems, which can cross medical specialties and make getting proper treatment extremely difficult.

Some autoimmune diseases cause chronic, consistent symptoms, while others are characterized by periods of remission (little or no disease activity) and flare (more disease activity). Autoimmune diseases commonly present with nonspecific symptoms like pain and fatigue, which are not easily identified with a particular condition and make diagnosis difficult. Symptoms can also vary widely from person to person,

making a correct diagnosis tough to nail down.

The symptoms of autoimmune disease can range from life-threatening and serious, rendering a patient in need of round-the-clock care, to a mild annoyance that barely disrupts a person's life. Most of us, however, fall in the middle of the spectrum—we live with chronic symptoms that impact our productivity and abilities, yet our healthcare providers and those in our support network often don't understand and are unable to provide lasting relief.

If you have an autoimmune disease, it's likely you will find the diagnosis process and treatment options challenging, at best. There is no medical specialty focusing on autoimmune disease in general. As a patient, you are treated by a specialist focused on the organ or system involved in the condition, rather than your whole body. If you are feeling isolated and lacking support, you are not alone—many of us have felt this way. If we have you worried, it's not all doom and gloom! There are ways of using the conventional system to your advantage and tools at your disposal for living well despite autoimmune disease.

WHAT TYPES OF AUTOIMMUNE DISEASES ARE THERE?

Autoimmune diseases are usually classified into two categories. There are organ-specific diseases, like Hashimoto's thyroiditis (which affects the thyroid gland) and type 1 diabetes (which affects the pancreas) and non-organ-specific diseases, like rheumatoid arthritis (which affects the joints) and lupus (which affects connective tissue). The most commonly affected organs are those of the endocrine system, such as the thyroid, pancreas, and adrenal glands. The most commonly affected non-organ tissues are those of the blood, like red blood cells, or connective tissue, like muscles and joints. Some diseases seem to occur between the two types and some people may experience several autoimmune diseases at the same time. Additionally, many autoimmune diseases commonly coexist with others, for example celiac disease and Hashimoto's thyroiditis. If you have three or more autoimmune diseases, you have multiple autoimmune syndrome.

The autoimmune process itself can also take different forms. Specific cells or tissues might steadily be damaged, an organ might grow excessively large, or the function of an organ may be disturbed. Some diseases are life threatening, others are disabling, and still others, if they are recognized early, can be successfully treated or managed relatively easily.

WHAT ARE THE RISKS FOR AND CAUSES OF AUTOIMMUNE DISEASE?

Autoimmune disease affects millions of Americans and many more people worldwide, but there are particular groups who are most at risk. In addition, research has identified three contributing factors that

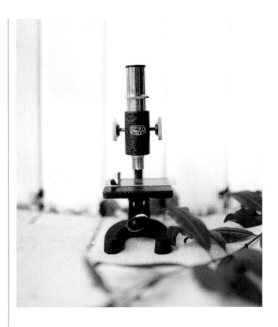

interact with each other to cause the development of autoimmune disease.

1. GENETICS—The genes you inherit from your parents play a part in determining your predisposition for developing an autoimmune disease, and because of this, it is very common for them to run in families. For instance, the incidence of celiac disease in the general population is 1 in 100 people, while the incidence in those with a first-degree family member who has it, like parents, siblings, or children, is 1 in 22.

Unlike genetic diseases, however, where one or two gene mutations are responsible for the disease, there are countless genes that affect your risk for autoimmune disease. Instead of inheriting one specific autoimmune gene, you inherit a larger collection that puts you at risk for developing an autoimmune disease. This may place you at more or less risk for certain diseases and it is why specific diseases are not always inherited in families, but many members of the same family suffer from different *related* autoimmune diseases. For instance, your mom may have type 1 diabetes, while your aunt has Crohn's, and your sister has Hashimoto's thyroiditis. Similarly, those who already have an autoimmune disease are at a higher risk for developing additional diseases, because they most likely have acquired the collection of genes that predisposes them to autoimmune disease.

Disproportionately 1 of the greatest risk factors is gender, with females making up 75 percent of the diagnosed autoimmune population, most likely because of the hormonal differences between the sexes. Your ethnicity is also a factor. African-Americans, Native Americans, and Latinos are at a greater risk than Caucasians.

2. ENVIRONMENTAL TRIGGERS—Although it can be handy to blame autoimmune disease all on genetics, it only accounts for about one-third of your risk of developing one. It is often said that while genes load the gun, environment pulls the trigger. Pathogens, chemicals, and substances your immune system is exposed to in your daily life can have an impact on whether or not you develop an autoimmune disease.

Certain bacterial and viral infections, both acute and chronic, have been linked to the development of autoimmunity—most likely because they contain proteins that closely resemble your own, confusing the immune system. Exposure to toxins and chemicals can similarly trigger autoimmunity. You are exposed to these components through pollution, the water supply, pesticides and herbicides in foods, cleaning products, personal-care products, chemical exposure in your home or in your workplace, and more.

3. DIET AND LIFESTYLE—A poor diet contributes to the development of autoimmune disease by exacerbating intestinal permeability, creating nutrient deficiencies, and overactivating the immune system. Similarly, sleep issues, lack of movement, and drug exposure, both prescription and recreational, can also increase your risk of developing autoimmune disease.

Stress also plays an important part in the autoimmune disease process. People experiencing acute and unmanaged stress or chronic stress are often at higher risk for developing autoimmune disease.

Finally, your geographic location may play a role. For example, in the United States, it has been shown that those living in the Pacific Northwest have a higher incidence of certain autoimmune diseases, which may be in part due to lack of natural sunlight at higher latitudes, contributing to vitamin D deficiency.

While you can't do much about your genetic inheritance and exposure to infectious disease, you *can* do something about managing your dietary and lifestyle choices, as well as limiting your contact with toxins and chemicals, and we'll get into this in more depth in Chapters 3 and 6.

DOES HAVING ONE AUTOIMMUNE DISEASE PUT YOU AT RISK FOR DEVELOPING OTHERS?

Roughly 25 percent of those of us with 1 autoimmune disease will go on to develop additional autoimmune diseases. Having 3 or more diagnosed autoimmune diseases is classified as multiple autoimmune syndrome (MAS). This syndrome usually includes one skin disorder, such as psoriasis or vitiligo. Awareness of the autoimmune diseases related to your current diagnosis can be helpful if signs of new diseases become apparent, as it can make these new diagnoses easier for health-care providers by pointing them toward likely disorders and allowing for earlier identification of multiple autoimmune syndrome. For instance, celiac disease is associated with type 1 diabetes, Hashimoto's thyroiditis, Graves' disease, and Addison's disease. Delay in diagnosis allows more time for further autoimmune diseases to develop, which is a second reason that awareness of MAS is so important.

(continued on page 8)

ANGIE'S EXPERIENCE

I have multiple autoimmune syndrome (MAS), which is defined as having three or more diagnosed autoimmune diseases. Mine are celiac disease, endometriosis, and lichen sclerosus. Lichen sclerosus (LS) is an autoimmune skin condition, and due to its nature (affecting the genitals and causing discomfort, tearing, and bruising of the skin), most sufferers are incredibly private about their diagnosis. When I received mine, I had no idea that it was an autoimmune disease, that my risks of developing further autoimmune diseases were heightened, or that MAS existed and how it often includes a skin condition. LS was my very first autoimmune diagnosis, and I learned about it many years before my next. Had I understood and been fully informed, perhaps I could have taken more preventative measures in my health care or proactively advocated for myself with doctors in order to be vigilant about developing new diseases. I might have even discovered the new diseases more quickly, if I had been able to point out my existing condition as autoimmune and help direct my doctor's suspicions as I grew more ill with autoimmune disease. I decided several years ago to begin speaking about LS publicly in the hope that others would feel less ashamed in seeking treatment for skin conditions, even ones that were difficult to reveal, in order to catch disease progression early and possibly prevent going on to develop additional autoimmune diseases.

LIST OF CONFIRMED AUTOIMMUNE, SUSPECTED AUTOIMMUNE, AND AUTOIMMUNE-RELATED CONDITIONS

While some diseases have a clear autoimmune component, many are *suspected* to have an autoimmune component, and in some cases, that has yet to be proven. Other conditions are known to be pathogenic in origin, but the initial infection can trigger an autoimmune response (such as Lyme or Chagas disease). We've compiled this list to include all conditions on the autoimmune spectrum ranging from specifically autoimmune to those that are suspected to be autoimmune in nature.

Acute disseminated encephalomyelitis (ADEM)

Acute necrotizing hemorrhagic leukoencephalitis (AHL)

Addison's disease

Agammaglobulinemia

Alopecia areata (AA)

Amyloidosis

Ankylosing spondylitis

Anti-GBM/Anti-TBM nephritis

Antiphospholipid syndrome (APS)

Autoimmune angioedema

Autoimmune aplastic anemia

Autoimmune dysautonomia

Autoimmune hemolytic anemia (AIHA)

Autoimmune hepatitis (AIH)

Autoimmune hyperlipidemia (AIH)

Autoimmune immunodeficiency

Autoimmune inner ear disease (AIED)

Autoimmune myocarditis

Autoimmune oophoritis

Autoimmune pancreatitis (AIP)

Autoimmune retinopathy (AIR)

Autoimmune thrombocytopenic purpura (ATP)

Autoimmune urticaria

Axonal and neuronal neuropathies

Balo disease

Behcet's disease

Bullous pemphigoid

Castleman's disease (CD)

Celiac disease

Chagas disease

Chronic inflammatory demyelinating polyneuropathy (CIDP)

Chronic recurrent multifocal osteomyelitis (CRMO)

Churg-Strauss syndrome (CSS)

Cicatricial pemphigoid/benign mucosal pemphigoid (MMP)

Cogan syndrome

Cold agglutinin disease

Congenital heart block

Coxsackie myocarditis

CREST syndrome

Crohn's disease

Dermatitis herpetiformis (DH)

Dermatomyositis (DM)

Devic's disease/neuromyelitis optica (NMO)

Discoid lupus

Dressler's syndrome

Endometriosis

Eosinophilic esophagitis (EoE)

Eosinophilic fasciitis (EF)

Erythema nodosum (EN)

Essential mixed cryoglobulinemia

Evans syndrome

Experimental allergic encephalomyelitis (AEA)

Fibrosing alveolitis

Giant cell arteritis/temporal arteritis (GCA)

Giant cell myocarditis

Glomerulonephritis

Goodpasture syndrome

Granulomatosis with polyangiitis (GPA) (formerly called Wegener's granulomatosis)

Graves' disease

Guillain-Barré syndrome (GBS)

Hashimoto's encephalopathy (HE)

Hashimoto's thyroiditis

Henoch-Schönlein purpura (HSP)

Herpes gestationis

Hypogammaglobulinemia

Idiopathic pulmonary fibrosis (IPF)

Idiopathic thrombocytopenic purpura (ITP)

IgA nephropathy

IgG4-related sclerosing disease

Inclusion body myositis (IBM)

Interstitial cystitis (IC)

Juvenile arthritis (JA)

Juvenile diabetes (type 1 diabetes)

Juvenile myositis (JM)

Kawasaki syndrome

Lambert-Eaton myasthenic syndrome

Leukocytoclastic vasculitis (LCV)

Lichen planus

Lichen sclerosus

Ligneous conjunctivitis (LC)

Linear IgA disease (LAD)

Lyme disease, chronic

Mèniére's disease

Microscopic polyangiitis (MPA)

Mixed connective tissue disease (MCTD)

Mooren's ulcer (MU)

Mucha-Habermann disease

Multiple sclerosis (MS)

Myasthenia gravis

Myositis

Narcolepsy

Neonatal lupus

Neutropenia

Ocular cicatricial pemphigoid (OCP)

Optic neuritis (ON)

Ord's thyroiditis

Palindromic rheumatism (PR)

Paraneoplastic cerebellar degeneration (PCD)

Paroxysmal nocturnal hemoglobinuria (PNH)

Parry-Romberg syndrome

Parsonage-Turner syndrome (PTS)

Pars planitis (peripheral uveitis)

Pediatric Autoimmune Neuropsychiatric Disorders Associated with Streptococcus (PANDAS)

Pemphigus vulgaris

Peripheral neuropathy

Perivenous encephalomyelitis

Pernicious anemia

POEMS syndrome

Polyarteritis nodosa (PAN)

Polymyalgia rheumatica (PMR)

Polymyositis (PM)

Postpericardiotomy syndrome (PPS)

Primary biliary cirrhosis (PBC)

Primary sclerosing cholangitis (PSC)

Psoriasis

Psoriatic arthritis

Pure red cell aplasia (PRCA)

Pyoderma gangrenosum

Raynaud's disease

Reactive arthritis/Reiter's syndrome

Reflex sympathetic dystrophy (RSD)

Relapsing polychondritis (RP)

Restless legs syndrome (RLS)

Retroperitoneal fibrosis (RPF)

Rheumatic fever

Rheumatoid arthritis (RA)

Sarcoidosis

Schmidt syndrome

Scleritis

Scleroderma

Sjögren's disease

Sperm and testicular autoimmunity

Stiff person syndrome (SPS)

Subacute bacterial endocarditis (SBE)

Susac's syndrome

Sympathetic ophthalmia (SO)

Systemic lupus erythematosus (SLE)

Takayasu's arteritis

Temporal arteritis/Giant cell arteritis (GCA)

Thrombocytopenic purpura (TTP)

Tolosa-Hunt syndrome (THS)

Transverse myelitis

Type 1 diabetes

Type 1, 2, and 3 polyglandular autoimmune syndromes (PAS)

Ulcerative colitis (UC)

Undifferentiated connective tissue disease (UCTD)

Uveitis

Vasculitis

Vesiculobullous dermatosis

Vitiligo

SEEKING DIAGNOSIS

Why Do You Need a Diagnosis?

In order to prevent complications from the damage caused by autoimmune disease, early diagnosis is essential. A correct diagnosis helps you to connect with the specialists and other medical providers you need, weigh treatment options, and think about how you want to navigate dietary and lifestyle modifications. Unfortunately, obtaining a proper diagnosis is often the *most* difficult part of the process for those of us suffering from autoimmune disease.

According to the American Autoimmune Related Diseases Association (AARDA), those with an autoimmune disease spend an average of 4 years seeking diagnosis, with visits to more than 4 physicians in the process. Some go undiagnosed for years, while others get misdiagnosed with other conditions. The undiagnosed and misdiagnosed rate for just 1 of these diseases, celiac disease, can be as high as 83 percent, which shows how difficult it truly can be to obtain answers. Autoimmune disease symptoms can be nonspecific, mild, and gradually build over time, making it difficult for you to determine if you need to see your physician about them. Often, when you do, you are told everything is fine and further testing that could uncover early warning signs isn't ordered.

One of the biggest issues with the treatment of autoimmune disease is that there is no medical specialty to serve these diseases as a whole. In combination with them being poorly understood by the medical profession, in general, this leads to patients being bounced around between primary-care physicians and specialists before obtaining proper testing and treatment. An AARDA study showed that 46 percent of autoimmune patients were told they were complainers or too obsessed with their health, instead of being offered the medical testing and treatment they needed.

Many of us who suffer from autoimmune symptoms wonder why we should even bother seeking a diagnosis, especially if our symptoms can improve just by making dietary and lifestyle changes. However, as you can see from the following list, there are benefits to having a clear diagnosis.

The benefits of having a diagnosis

1. It helps you connect with the right medical specialist for your condition.

2. It helps medical practitioners decide which testing to pursue regularly to gauge progress.

3. It helps you and your doctor decide which treatment option (medication, surgical, or other) is best for you.

4. It helps you connect with others who are suffering from the same condition.

5. It helps complementary care practitioners tailor their programs and protocols specifically to your needs.

6. It enables you to research and educate yourself about your disease.

(continued on page 12)

WHERE ARE YOU ON THE SPECTRUM?

Autoimmune Status Self-Test

You cannot get anywhere if you don't know your starting point. We've designed this test to help you evaluate where you are right now. Think of it like the big map in the center of the mall stating, "You are here." The point is not to dwell on your current experience, but to inform you about where you want to go next in terms of diagnosis, treatment, and lifestyle changes.

We were inspired by the idea that autoimmune disease often occurs on a spectrum, instead of being black or white (first talked about by Amy Myers, MD, in *The Autoimmune Solution*), as well as the ideas of Datis Kharrazian, DC, regarding "silent autoimmunity." This test blends their material with our experience in order to empower those who are suffering from autoimmune disease or chronic illness by providing a starting point.

INSTRUCTIONS: You will find two sections, the first with the same scoring for each question, and the second with an individual scoring system per question. At the end of the test, you will add the scores from both sections to come up with your **AUTOIMMUNE STATUS**. From there, you will have some information to guide the next steps in your healing journey. You can also come back to Section 1 of this test once you have made some changes to gauge your healing progress over time.

SECTION 1

Mark the blank with the number that best corresponds to how frequently you experience that symptom.

SCORING

0 = never occurs

1 = occurs rarely (monthly)

2 = occurs occasionally (weekly)

3 = occurs frequently (daily)

____ Fatigue and lack of energy

____ Chronic pain—muscles, joints, and bones

____ Heaviness in limbs, loss of muscle tone

____ Morning stiffness

____ Weakness and/or tremor

____ Headaches

____ Feeling puffy or inflamed

____ Rashes, hives, and skin issues of unknown origin

____ Dry eyes, mouth, or skin

____ Dermatitis or itchy skin

____ White patches on skin or inside of the mouth

____ Mouth ulcers

____ Trouble maintaining a healthy weight

____ Difficulty with exercise

____ IBS, or irritable bowel syndrome—constipation, diarrhea, or both

____ Abdominal pain or stomach cramps

____ Blood or mucus in stool

____ Trouble falling or staying asleep

____ Cold hands or feet and trouble staying warm

____ Heat intolerance and/or sun sensitivity

____ Rapid heartbeat

____ Night sweats

____ Difficulty swallowing, hoarseness, or lump in the throat

____ Decreased sense of taste or smell

____ Difficulty concentrating or focusing (brain fog)

____ Thinning hair or hair loss

____ Loss of outer third of eyebrow

____ Numbness or tingling in extremities

____ Dizziness or lightheadedness

____ Food allergies/sensitivities

____ Dark circles under eyes

____ Unexplained low-grade fever

____ Periodontal infections or gum issues

____ **TOTAL FOR SECTION 1**
(keep this handy to add below)

SECTION 2

This section is scored a little differently—follow the instructions on each question and total them at the bottom.

WOMEN ONLY

____ I am a woman **(0 = no, 10 = yes)**

____ My period is heavy and I cannot make it through without disruptive pain. **(0 = no, 1 = yes)**

____ Infertility **(0 = no, 1 = yes)**

____ Multiple miscarriages **(0 = no, 1 = yes)**

EVERYONE

____ Anemia of any type **(0 = no, 1 = yes)**

____ Osteoporosis or osteopenia **(0 = no, 1 = yes)**

____ History of chronic viral condition (Epstein-Barr, mono, herpes, shingles, chronic fatigue syndrome, hepatitis, or other chronic viral condition) **(0 = no, 5 = yes)**

____ A doctor has told me I was too sensitive. **(0 = no, 5 = yes)**

____ Members of my immediate family have autoimmune conditions **(0 = no, 5 = one, 10 = more than one)**

ANSWER ONE OF THE FOLLOWING, IF IT APPLIES TO YOU

____ I have a diagnosis of one autoimmune disease. **(0 = no, 30 = yes)**

____ I have a diagnosis of two autoimmune diseases. **(0 = no, 40 = yes, in addition to the previous question)**

____ I have a diagnosis of three or more autoimmune diseases. **(0 = no, 50 = yes, in addition to the previous two questions)**

____ **TOTAL FOR SECTION 2**

Now add up the values from Section 1 and Section 2 to discover your autoimmune status.

___ **SECTION 1 TOTAL** + ___ **SECTION 2 TOTAL** = ___ **YOUR AUTOIMMUNE STATUS**

Compare your autoimmune status score with the categories below:

SCORING

1-29, STATUS 1: It appears your risk for having an autoimmune disease is low, however if some of the symptoms you are experiencing are bothersome, you should make it a priority to speak with your doctor to find out if they could be caused by other conditions.

30-59, STATUS 2: It appears your risk for having an autoimmune disease is average. This is the phase practitioners sometimes refer to as "silent autoimmunity." This means that there may be antibodies present, but you are not experiencing disruptive symptoms. If you are suffering from autoimmune disease, this is the best time to seek diagnosis and take action although it can be difficult because many symptoms are not yet present so your doctor may not agree to order antibody testing. If you are having trouble working with your health-care providers on this, we provide more insight in Chapter 2.

60-99, STATUS 3: It appears your risk for having an autoimmune disease is high, and it is possible that some of your symptoms could be caused by

an autoimmune reaction. However, seeking diagnosis may be difficult—although symptoms are present, they might not point to a clear diagnosis. Intervention at this status can significantly improve your quality of life.

100+, STATUS 4: You've been diagnosed with an autoimmune disease already, or your combination of health history and current symptoms make diagnosis very likely. Diagnosis at this stage is usually quick, due to multiple and clear symptoms pointing to a specific disease. It is necessary to form a health-care team (if you don't already have one), start treatment, and consider changes immediately in order to regain quality of life.

WHAT TO DO WITH THIS INFORMATION

Don't get derailed by the specifics of your symptoms or your autoimmune status according to this test—instead, use this information as a starting point for conversations with your health-care team. In Chapter 2, we will give you suggestions on how to assemble this team and quickly move forward with plans to restore your best health.

7. It helps you and your doctor practice good preventative care, order testing to gauge progress, and anticipate potential issues.

8. It helps you understand what disease progression might look like as well as signs and symptoms to be aware of.

9. It gives you peace of mind knowing what is causing your symptoms.

What If You Can't Get a Diagnosis?

Sometimes patients suffer from chronic symptoms that could be autoimmune in nature but can't obtain a diagnosis for one reason or another. This might be because of poor-quality medical care or a lack of access to medical care, lack of financial resources for medical care, or not being able to find a collaborative physician who is willing to do the proper testing to make a diagnosis. If you find yourself in this situation, don't fret! We give you lots of information about how to find a collaborative health-care provider who can assist you in Chapter 2.

Overlapping Diagnoses

It is common for someone who has one autoimmune disease already to get a diagnosis of additional autoimmune diseases during his or her lifetime. Adding to this, symptoms of some autoimmune conditions are often similar to others, which is known as overlap. This occurs most in the autoimmune conditions that affect connective tissue, such as rheumatoid arthritis, scleroderma, Raynaud's disease, mixed connective tissue disease, Sjögren's disease, and lupus. Some autoimmune conditions frequently coexist with others, like Hashimoto's thyroiditis and Graves' disease.

These symptom and disease overlaps can make it difficult to obtain an accurate diagnosis and proper treatment. Patients with multiple autoimmune conditions often see different specialists to manage each one. In the case of multiple autoimmune diagnoses, the disease with the most severe symptoms is usually given treatment preference. If you find yourself here, make sure that you are connected to providers who are well equipped to track all of your conditions, even the ones that may not be causing the most severe symptoms.

Common Misdiagnoses

Because autoimmune disease can cause nonspecific symptoms that overlap with many conditions, patients can often be misdiagnosed with other, nonautoimmune conditions, or they may not be suffering from an autoimmune condition in the first place. It is important to be aware of these diseases that can produce similar symptoms, in addition to the fact that a person can suffer from autoimmune disease in combination with other nonautoimmune conditions.

Here is a list of conditions that are commonly confused with autoimmune disease.

- Alzheimer's or Parkinson's disease
- Chronic fatigue syndrome (CFS)

- Chronic infection (can trigger autoimmunity)
- Fibromyalgia
- Irritable bowel syndrome (IBS)
- Lyme disease (can result in autoimmunity)
- Mental disorders like depression, anxiety, and bipolar disorder
- Migraines
- Nutrient deficiency (like anemia)
- Sleep apnea

How do you know if you have been misdiagnosed? This can be tricky to pinpoint and involves a lot of trial and error, but most people find that one or all of the following is true: They do not improve using the typical treatments for their disease; they begin to experience symptoms not explained by their diagnosis; or they continue to get tested and uncover a new diagnosis. For example, a common misdiagnosis for celiac disease is IBS, and patients may realize it was a misdiagnosis when they do not respond to the common IBS treatment.

How Do You Cope with a Diagnosis?

Although at first it can seem rather cut and dry to receive an autoimmune disease diagnosis, it is rarely that simple. Most of us experience a range of complex emotions following diagnosis. Often the initial reaction is one of relief; you may feel grateful to know the cause of previously unexplained symptoms. This is especially true with an autoimmune diagnosis, since the disease may have been progressing for years with confusing periods of illness and remission that are often dismissed by family, friends, and even physicians. A diagnosis can offer you much-needed validation.

It is not uncommon for your relief to quickly fade, though, and for you to enter the grieving process. Many of us with autoimmune disease encounter a tremendous loss of identity prior to and following diagnosis and may experience some or all of the emotions associated with the Kübler-Ross stages of grief, including denial, anger, bargaining, depression, and acceptance. This process is not necessarily linear, and you might find yourself going back and forth through some of these emotions as you come to terms with your disease.

Many autoimmune disease sufferers report feeling that they are alone and not understood by others. You may struggle to construct a new sense of self, which may be difficult for your loved ones to accept. The ability of your family and friends to cope well with the diagnosis itself may also be very difficult, leading to an even greater sense of isolation. Further, you may experience profound anxiety about increasing physical disability, reliance on others, hospitalizations, treatment options, pain levels, financial strain of health-care costs, and your ability to maintain a job. Understandably, the feeling of being alone coupled with very real physical, emotional, and social concerns can lead to depression.

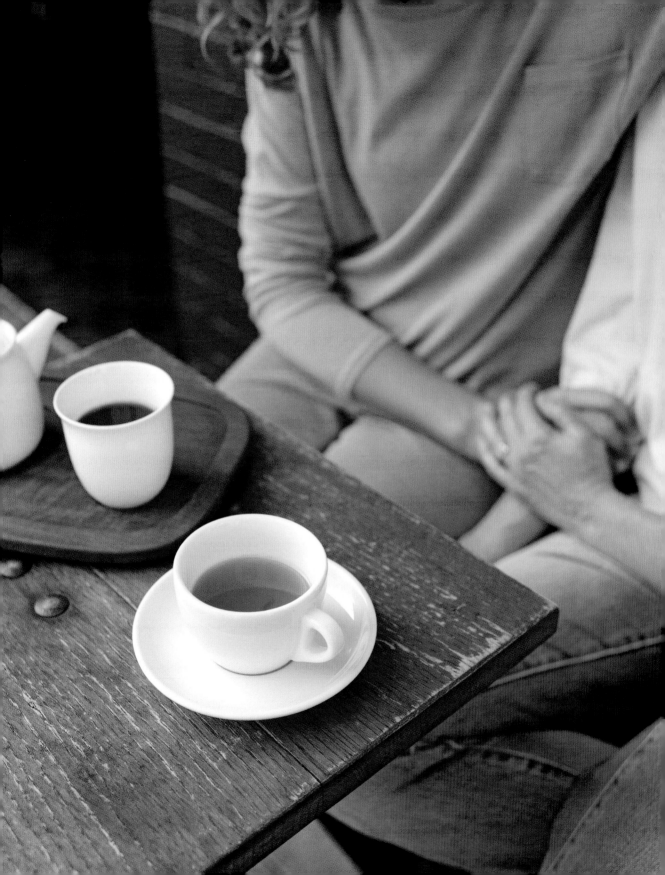

However, most of us suffering from autoimmune disease can successfully navigate the grieving process and overcome any diagnosis-related depression, eventually finding even greater happiness and personal depth. This requires learning the skills associated with resilience.

For you to rebound successfully after receiving a life-changing autoimmune diagnosis, you need to learn to be resilient. Resilience is a set of skills that gives us the ability to withstand stress and adversity. The first and most important thing to understand about resilience is that it is not something we are born with, and it is not a personality trait. Again, it is a set of skills, which *can* be learned and, with practice, better used.

Practicing Resilience

Resilience comes down to six behaviors. Taking these actions repeatedly, even if they do not come naturally to you, allows resilience to build.

- **MAINTAINING A POSITIVE SELF-IMAGE**—having confidence in your strengths and abilities and viewing yourself as a survivor, rather than as a victim.

- **MANAGING EMOTIONS AND IMPULSES**—this means not freaking out. Although a crisis may at first seem overwhelming, taking time to adjust yourself and then reacting in a calm, composed manner is more effective than losing it.

- **TAKING CHARGE OF THINGS IN YOUR CONTROL**—actively problem solving, communicating clearly with those around you, and seeking resources that can help you.

- **ESTABLISHING HEALTHY VERSUS HARMFUL COPING STRATEGIES**—finding ways to laugh, getting exercise, practicing prayer or meditation, considering talk therapy, if appropriate, or spending time with loved ones versus harmful strategies like abusing alcohol or drugs.

- **INVESTING IN CLOSE RELATIONSHIPS**—forming intimate personal relationships if you are lacking them or devoting time to the important ones that already exist. These relationships together function as a crucial support system that allows you to ask for help and give help. The "giving help" part matters as much as the "getting help," because it increases meaning in your own life.

- **FINDING POSITIVE MEANING IN LIFE EVENTS**—reframing negative situations to see their value or the favorable effects these situations may have had on you as a person.

Don't allow your diagnosis to discourage you; instead, incorporate resilience into your response to the new information you've received. This crucial information allows you to move toward wellness.

LEARN ABOUT YOUR CONDITION

Testing

There are many laboratory tests that are used to diagnose or gauge treatment progress for those with autoimmune diseases. Depending on your diagnosis or symptoms, you may undergo certain testing only for diagnosis and then another set of testing regularly to assess disease progression and treatment results. These can be divided into four categories.

1. ANTIBODY TESTS—Testing for both antinuclear and autoantibodies is common if there is a known test for the particular autoimmune disease. These tests tell the doctor which tissues the body is targeting and at what rate. Most of the time, antibodies can be directed at the self (tissues within the body), but other times they can be directed toward environmental triggers, such as in the case of transglutaminase (a protein found in wheat) in celiac disease. Antibody tests are used by specialists to make a diagnosis and determine treatment, as well as to gauge how that treatment is working for you.

The following are some common antibody blood tests.

- **ANTINUCLEAR ANTIBODIES (ANA)**—These are antibodies that target the nucleus of a cell. Sometimes they are present in autoimmune diseases that affect connective tissue, such as systemic lupus erythematosus, Sjögren's disease, and mixed connective tissue disease. It is important to note that sometimes a positive ANA is found in people without autoimmune disease, and further evaluation is needed for a doctor to make a diagnosis.

- **RHEUMATOID FACTOR**—This is an antibody that is commonly found in autoimmune diseases that affect the joints, like rheumatoid arthritis.

- **THYROID ANTIBODIES** (TPO, TgAB, and TSI)—These are three antibody tests that are commonly used to diagnose and treat autoimmune thyroid conditions like Hashimoto's and Graves' disease.

- **ANTITRANSGLUTAMINASE ANTIBODIES**—This

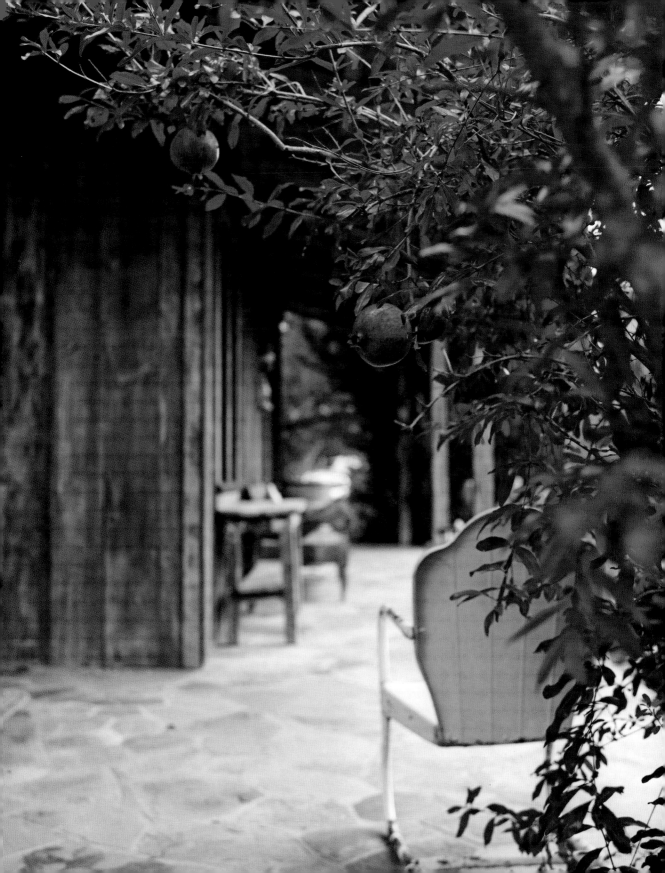

test indicates antibodies to proteins found in gluten, which are found in those with celiac disease.

2. TESTING TO DETERMINE ORGAN DAMAGE AND/OR INFLAMMATION—These tests are related to whichever organ is affected by your diagnosed or suspected autoimmune disease. They range from minimally invasive (such as a thyroid ultrasound) to more invasive (such as a colonoscopy). Sometimes the tests are only needed to make a diagnosis, and other times, they are repeated to gauge your progress or to make ongoing decisions about treatment.

Here are some common tests and procedures.

- **UPPER ENDOSCOPY**—This is a procedure where a small camera on a flexible tube is used to visually examine your esophagus, stomach, and duodenum (beginning of the small intestine). It may also be used to collect tissue samples for a biopsy. This procedure is used in the diagnosis and treatment of diseases affecting the upper gastrointestinal system, like celiac disease.

- **COLONOSCOPY**—This is a procedure where a small camera on a flexible tube is used to visually examine your colon and rectum. It may also be used to collect tissue samples for a biopsy. This procedure is used in the diagnosis and treatment of diseases affecting the lower gastrointestinal system, like Crohn's disease and ulcerative colitis.

- **MAGNETIC RESONANCE IMAGING (MRI)**— This is a test where you are placed in a tube-shaped machine that contains magnets that move back and forth. The magnetic field created by this movement, as well as radio waves, creates detailed cross-section images of tissues throughout your body. This test is used in the diagnosis and treatment of diseases such as multiple sclerosis.

- **X-RAY**—This is a test where a picture is made of the internal structures of your body, where dense materials such as bone show up well. This test is used in the diagnosis and treatment of diseases that affect the joints and connective tissue, such as rheumatoid arthritis, systemic lupus erythematosus, and mixed connective tissue disease.

- **ULTRASOUND**—This is a test that uses high-frequency sound waves to produce images within your body. It is used in the diagnosis and treatment of diseases that affect certain organs, like the thyroid in Hashimoto's disease.

3. GENERAL TESTING RELATED TO OVERALL HEALTH—This testing ranges from being specifically related to the known process of an autoimmune disease (such as the malabsorption of iron and vitamin B_{12} that is a known factor in celiac disease) to just checking up on your overall well-being and making sure that all organs are functioning properly.

Here are some common general tests.

- **CBC (COMPLETE BLOOD COUNT)**—This is an overall blood test screen that will reveal things like anemia, infection, and blood disorders.

- **CMP (COMPREHENSIVE METABOLIC PANEL)**—This is a broad screening to evaluate liver and kidney function that is particularly of interest to those on certain medications.

- **NUTRITIONAL ANEMIA PROFILE**—These are a series of blood tests including hemoglobin, hematocrit, folate, ferritin, and B_{12} that helps find the source and track the progress of anemia, which is a common symptom of many autoimmune diseases.

- **VITAMIN AND MINERAL TESTS**—These are specific blood tests that look for deficiencies in certain vitamins and minerals and are sometimes performed in conjunction with other panels (such as a CMP). Common tests include vitamin B_{12}, vitamin D, and iron.

- **CRP (C-REACTIVE PROTEIN) AND ESR (ERYTHROCYTE SEDIMENTATION RATE)**—These are blood tests that indicate the level of inflammation in your body and are useful for tracking treatment progress in conditions like rheumatoid arthritis.

- **LIPID PROFILE**—This is a collection of blood tests that look at the amount of cholesterol and triglycerides in your blood.

- **THYROID PANEL**—This is a collection of blood tests that look at the amount of thyroid hormones in your blood. It is common to include TSH (thyroid stimulating hormone) and total T4; sometimes "free" T3, "free" T4, as well as reverse T3 and antibody tests are included.

4. FUNCTIONAL MEDICINE TESTING—While not common, those patients working with a functional medicine practitioner may have testing ordered that goes beyond what is standard in the conventional medical system. These tests are not needed for diagnosis but can help guide your treatment when considering a holistic approach.

- **COMPREHENSIVE STOOL TESTING**—To perform this test, you send a stool sample to a lab to be evaluated for pathogenic overgrowths or infections like bacteria, yeast, and parasites. Some stool tests include testing pathogens against potential antimicrobial agents, both prescription and herbal, which can be incredibly helpful for guiding your treatment.

- **HORMONE TESTING**—This is a salivary test used to determine your hormonal balance, both for sex and stress hormones. Many tests call for multiple samples, providing a complete picture of how your levels are fluctuating over a period of time.

- **MICRONUTRIENT TESTING**—This is a blood test that can help determine if you have any micronutrient deficiencies that aren't picked up on a conventional lab test (such as vitamin A or selenium).

- **GENETIC TESTING**—These are both blood and saliva tests that help determine if you have a genetic mutation that may predispose you to autoimmune disease (such as the HLA-DQ gene mutations, as well as the MTHFR gene mutations).

- **FOOD AND ENVIRONMENTAL ALLERGEN TESTING**—These are blood tests that help determine if you have any sensitivities to food or environmental triggers and can help determine personalized diet and lifestyle interventions.

- **ORGANIC ACIDS TESTING**—This is a urine test that can help pinpoint metabolic issues, pathogenic overgrowths, neurotransmitter imbalance, oxidative stress, and impaired methylation.

- **HEAVY METALS TESTING**—This is a test that is performed by drinking a chelating agent (a substance that helps draw out minerals) and then taking a urine sample. It is used to determine if you have a high load of heavy metals in your body.

What Is the Treatment for Autoimmune Disease?

Unfortunately, there is no cure for autoimmune disease—once the immune system starts attacking the body's own tissues, there is nothing that can be done to get it to "turn off" or stop the attack. Current conventional treatment is focused on slowing inflammation, preserving organs, and managing symptoms. At best, this treatment has you barely putting a dent in your symptoms while creating a whole lot of side effects.

Patients going through this experience often find themselves frustrated. Some are told there is nothing that can be done, finding themselves with mild but irritating symptoms that don't warrant powerful medications. Others find themselves on immunosuppressants and then have to suffer or worry about side effects like infection or cancer. Those with even more serious and life-threatening flares or conditions may find themselves facing surgical intervention, although this is not typical.

The current approach to managing autoimmune disease isn't as hopeless as it seems! There is a burgeoning community of people reclaiming their health with a new approach. You will find some useful solutions integrating the best of conventional medicine with natural interventions throughout the rest of this book.

Common medical treatments for autoimmune diseases include:

- **NONSTEROIDAL ANTI-INFLAMMATORIES (NSAIDS)**—These are medications that reduce inflammation and relieve pain. They are available over-the-counter or by prescription and are used to treat muscle or joint stiffness and pain, aches, menstrual pain, and headaches. Many patients with joint pain, for example, use NSAIDs to manage it.

- **HORMONE REPLACEMENT**—In diseases that result in a loss of hormone (such as type 1 diabetes or Hashimoto's thyroiditis), replacement hormone (like insulin or levothyroxine) is usually prescribed.

- **CORTICOSTEROIDS**—These medications suppress inflammation by mimicking the body's own steroid hormones. They are prescribed in different forms and may be taken orally, topically, inhaled, and by injection. While effective, steroid medications can come with unpleasant side effects, like mood swings and weight gain.

- **ANTIBIOTICS**—Certain autoimmune conditions, such as ankylosing spondylitis, are linked to bacterial infections (in this case *Klebsiella pneumoniae*), for which antibiotics may be prescribed.

- **DISEASE-MODIFYING ANTIRHEUMATIC DRUGS (DMARDS)**—In conditions with more serious symptoms, these medications are used to suppress the immune system, thereby calming the autoimmune process. They are available orally or by injection and usually take weeks to months to start working. They are not risk-free, as suppressing the immune system can cause a greater susceptibility to infection as well as certain types of cancer. Additionally, these medications can be hard on the liver and kidneys.

- **BIOLOGIC DMARDS (ALSO CALLED TNF INHIBITORS)**—These are newer types of DMARDs made to mimic the activity of compounds in your body (hence the name biologic). They are available by injection, tend to be quicker acting, and are often prescribed in addition to traditional DMARDs. They carry a similar side effect risk as other DMARDs, with possibly a higher risk for infection because of the specific part of the immune system they suppress.

- **SURGERY**—Although this is not as common, some autoimmune diseases can result in surgical intervention, such as Crohn's disease, ulcerative colitis, and endometriosis.

In addition to these treatments specifically to control autoimmune disease, you may find yourself put on other medications to control the side effects. Not uncommon are medications that affect digestion, like antacids, proton-pump inhibitors, H2 blockers, laxatives, and antidiarrheals; antibiotics and antifungals to treat infections; and hormonal treatments.

Is There Anything Else You Can Do?

In this book, we are not proposing diet and lifestyle interventions as a treatment in and of itself for autoimmune disease; rather, we are suggesting that there are things you as an autoimmune patient can do for yourself *in addition to the medical treatment you receive from your practitioner or team* (with their blessing, of course!). Many autoimmune patients have regained their health using a combination of natural approaches and conventional medicine. It's not a matter of one or the other, but how everything works in concert to produce lasting wellness.

The following are some natural approaches that you may be able to incorporate in an effort to live healthier. We will be talking more in depth about each of these items, but brief descriptions are outlined below.

- **DIET**—Research has established a link between leaky gut (otherwise known as "intestinal permeability") and all autoimmune diseases. A dietary approach that: (1) provides all of the nutrients needed for optimal healing and recovery and (2) eliminates all food allergies and sensitivities is best for long-term healing and management (see Chapter 3).

- **SLEEP**—The inability to fall asleep, poor-quality sleep, or interrupted sleep are issues that many with chronic illness suffer from. Because sleep is necessary for proper hormonal balance as well as repair and restoration of the body, troubleshooting these barriers to proper sleep can make a big difference (see Chapter 4).

- **STRESS MANAGEMENT**—Chronic stress is well known to cause autoimmune flares because of its impact on the body's hormonal balance. Learning how to manage stress effectively and appropriately can help reduce this impact (see Chapter 5).

- **EXERCISE**—Improper movement or lack of movement can contribute negatively to autoimmune symptoms. It is important to engage in the right type of exercise at a difficulty level that is right for the circumstances (see Chapter 6).

- **SUPPORT**—Connecting with others and nature is an important part of the long-term management of chronic illness and autoimmune disease (see Chapter 7).

INFORMATION GATHERING

Organizing Medical Information

It is important for you to have all of your medical information and records on hand and organized so that they can be easily accessed. Those suffering from chronic illness tend to see a lot of new practitioners, and information can very easily get lost in the process. Having your own records on hand also gives you the opportunity to track changes over time. Follow these simple steps to make sure that you have your medical information organized so that it can best be used to guide your care.

1. Always request copies of your lab tests and documents while at your doctor's office. You have a right to have a copy of this information for your records. It is possible to request duplicate files of any imaging (MRI, CT scan, x-ray) and store them on a hard drive for long-term safekeeping.

2. Keep a file of medical information in a convenient location at home. If your records are digital, print copies in case the record is accidentally lost or destroyed. Organize by date for easy access, with one large folder for each year filled with files for each month. You can also consider using one of the many health-tracking apps on your mobile phone that can store photographed records and information and track lab result changes over time.

3. If you have a condition like hypothyroidism, where the same lab tests are performed on a regular basis, consider making a spreadsheet on your computer for easy comparison of lab values and to track changes over time. Again, an app may be useful for long-term tracking.

4. When bringing your own medical records to a new doctor or appointment, make copies and leave the originals at home so that the practitioner can keep them for his or her records. This way you always keep a complete record at home.

Keeping a Symptom Journal

Journaling is a tool that everyone can use to track progress while on a healing journey. The ways of keeping a journal are innumerable—you could use pen and paper, a word or text document on your computer, a spreadsheet, or an app on your smartphone. More important than the method you use is the fact that you actually do it in a consistent way where the data can be used to inform future decisions.

Metrics to track

- Energy
- Pain
- Bowel movements
- Exercise
- Mood
- Food/beverage intake (see Note, page 24)
- Notable symptoms
- Body measurements
- Digestion
- Medications
- Supplements
- Stress management

Tracking tips

- Use a scale from 1 to 10 instead of adjectives ("energy—7" instead of "I had a good amount of energy today"), making your data more usable. This will also make it quicker for you to track results and make them easy to compare.

- In order to avoid being overwhelmed, only track what is important. Start with a

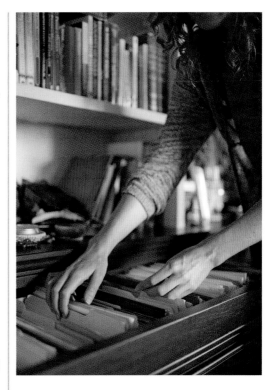

few metrics and build as you get into the habit.

- Don't beat yourself up if you get busy and forget a few days. Maintaining the record long-term is useful even if there are some gaps.

- Assess and track your bowel movements regularly to see if there are any changes due to your diet or lifestyle.

Once you are in the habit of regular tracking, set aside a time once a month to go over your journal and see if you can make any correlations. You may be able to put things together in a way you couldn't while in the moment— maybe you get bloated consistently after eating a certain food, or you notice that you had a headache every day since introducing a new supplement. Tracking becomes incredibly important anytime you incorporate something new into your routine—like a medication, supplement, exercise, or a food reintroduction (which we will talk more about on page 75).

Even if you are just beginning your healing journey, learning how to track sooner rather than later is a great idea. You may feel as though tracking now is not going to do any good since you don't have a plan, but it is always useful to have a baseline of how you were feeling before you started to make changes (just think how useful it will be for looking back on your progress!).

NOTE: We aren't suggesting to obsessively count food intake or weigh yourself every day, even if one of your goals is weight loss. When tracking food, describing the foods you ate that day (i.e., salad with carrots, lettuce, beets, canned salmon, and avocado dressing) in enough detail to make connections about diet and symptoms is more than good enough. Even if you would like to lose weight, we recommend ditching the scale (that number doesn't tell us anything about your value!) and relying on weekly body measurements instead. Actual calorie counting can be useful for up to a week just to see a ballpark range of how much food you are eating and to determine if all nutritional requirements are being met.

WHAT IS THE PROGNOSIS FOR AUTOIMMUNE DISEASES?

Each specific autoimmune disease has unpredictable outcomes. Some are aggressive and can be life-threatening, while others appear quickly, but spontaneously pass. Occasionally, autoimmune diseases can be both acute and chronic. Understanding which category your disease falls into can help you communicate better with your health-care providers.

Autoimmune disease is generally not an acute medical crisis, and it most likely manifests as a long-term, chronic illness. The course it will take in your body is uncertain and not something a doctor is capable of predicting for you. However, those of us with autoimmune disease can actively work to decrease factors that may worsen symptoms and strive to improve our prognosis. With a strong plan and health-care team in place, living well long-term is usually possible.

It is worth noting here that the Western health-care model is set up to excel in treatment of acute health crises, like a broken leg or a heart attack, but not necessarily of chronic illness—this is why personal advocacy is so important.

CALL TO ACTION

This first chapter was meant to do two things, convince you that knowledge is power on your autoimmune journey and provide you with some of the details that you should explore in order to get empowered. This basic information—what an autoimmune disease is, how to get a diagnosis, and the particulars to learn about your specific disease—is the foundation for transformation. Wellness is not in your doctor's office or in a new pill; it is in your hands, and it starts with being *informed*.

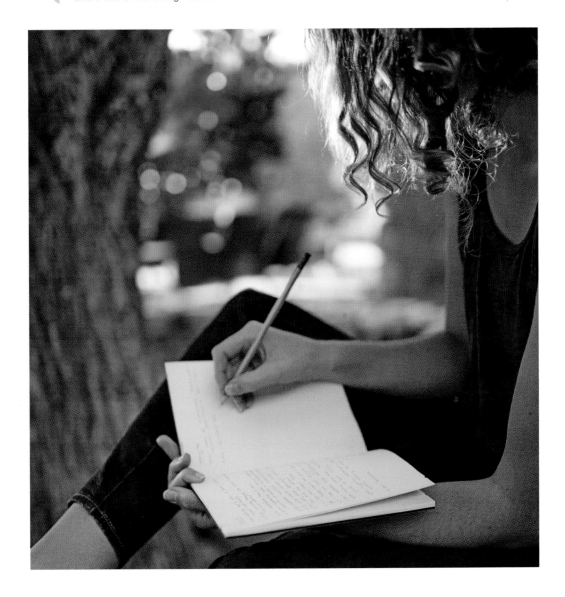

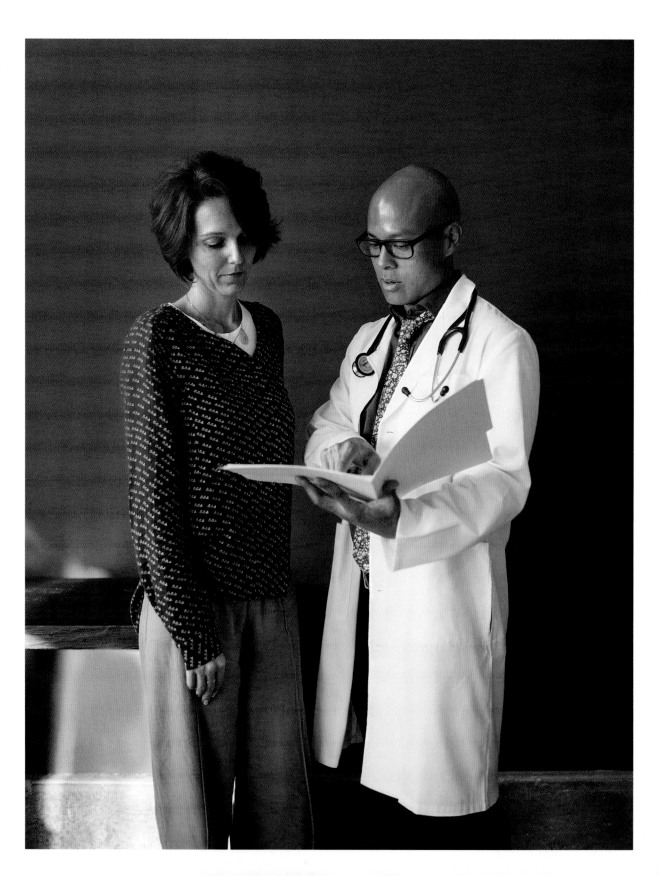

CHAPTER 2

Collaborate

"No one can whistle a symphony. It takes a whole orchestra to play it." —H. E. LUCCOCK

WE THINK THE SECOND MOST IMPORTANT thing you can do on your journey to wellness is to build a collaborative health-care team—a group of experts who advocate for and assist you with the medical and nonmedical aspects of healing. In this chapter, we'll be shedding some light on the different types of practitioners you can collaborate with, as well as give you some tips on assembling and managing your team. First, we need to answer the question of what collaboration truly means, especially as it applies to navigating the health-care system.

WHAT IS COLLABORATION?

Collaboration is one of those buzzwords without a widely agreed-upon definition. What we are using here is the integration of several definitions as they apply to managing your health-care team. Here is a further breakdown for more clarity.

- Collaboration is required in situations where you are not able to solve a problem on your own.

- Collaboration means openly sharing knowledge and being accountable, since actions taken by one member of your team can impact the others.

- Collaboration means blending what you and each member of your team can offer and combining the most useful ideas into one effective plan in order to best resolve a problem.

With that clear understanding of the concept, it becomes obvious to those of us with autoimmune disease that collaboration is absolutely necessary for the best possible treatment. Unquestionably, it is vital in the case of complex and changing medical situations, such as chronic illness and autoimmune disease, to take a collaborative approach. Unfortunately, collaboration between medical specialties within the conventional system, let alone with other types of alternative and complementary care providers, is rare.

It is up to you to advocate for a collaborative approach to your care and to build a team of providers who will share that cooperative vision. Luckily, we've clarified every aspect of that process for you in the following pages. Let's start by looking at the different types of health-care approaches and the different types of providers you may want to include on your team.

NATURAL VERSUS CONVENTIONAL MEDICAL APPROACHES

What Kinds of Practitioners Are There?

There are many practitioners with various backgrounds and training that can guide and assist you on your journey back to health. It is important to educate yourself about the many different types of licenses and specialties your practitioners may have so that you make the absolute best choice for your needs. The need for a doctor is not specific enough—what kind of doctor will best suit your situation? For example, if you have Hashimoto's thyroiditis, you may be best served by an endocrinologist, an integrative medical doctor (MD), or a naturopathic doctor (ND). Although all of these practitioners may be able to diagnose and treat your condition, the treatment they prescribe is going to be different, depending on their education and what kind of natural medicine, if any, they incorporate into their practice.

It is important to note which types of practitioners are licensed (which means they have met standards that qualify them to practice), which ones are medical (qualified to diagnose and treat), and which are nonlicensed and nonmedical. The latter type of practitioners can be vital assets to your health-care team, but you cannot expect to have your medical needs met through working with them. At the very least, you need to have a primary care provider, or a practitioner whom you see first for annual exams and when you are experiencing health problems. Depending on your insurance and where you live, this can be a medical doctor (MD), doctor of osteopathy (DO), nurse practitioner (NP), physician assistant (PA), or naturopathic doctor (ND).

Types of Licensed Conventional Medical Practitioners

These are practitioners who have gone through rigorous training to obtain their licenses to provide medical support, either at the highest level, such as a physician with a specialty, or at the supportive level, such as a registered nurse or dietician.

MEDICAL DOCTOR (MD)—a medical professional who has obtained a license to diagnose and treat medical conditions by completing medical school (generally 4 to 6 years after completing a bachelor's degree) as well as a residency (an internship lasting at least 2 years). They have to pass an exam to acquire state licenses. Most medical doctors either practice general care (internal medicine, family medicine, or pediatrics) or specialize in one system of the body.

DOCTOR OF OSTEOPATHIC MEDICINE (DO)— a medical professional who has received training that is very similar to that of an MD—medical school, residency, and an exam to obtain a license. Like an MD, he or she can choose any area of specialty or practice general care. The difference between the DO and MD training, however, is that a DO gets more emphasis on primary-care education, a whole-body approach, preventive care, the musculoskeletal system, and manipulative treatment.

Common medical specialties for both MD and DO include:

- Cardiology—heart
- Dermatology—skin
- Endocrinology—hormone and metabolic systems
- Gastroenterology—digestive tract
- Hematology—blood
- Immunology—immune system
- Nephrology—kidneys
- Obstetrics/gynecology—pregnancy and women's health
- Oncology—cancer
- Orthopedics—bone and connective tissue
- Otorhinolaryngology—ear, nose, and throat issues
- Psychiatry—emotional or mental illness
- Pulmonary—respiratory system
- Rheumatology—musculoskeletal issues

PHYSICIAN ASSISTANT (PA)— a health-care worker who practices medicine in partnership with medical doctors. Training takes 2 to 3 years to complete, much less than an MD, but is similar in scope. Thus, PAs are able to make health care more accessible and affordable by being able to see patients quicker and spend more time with them. A PA often works within a medical specialty just like an MD or DO.

REGISTERED NURSE (RN)— a general health-care worker who specializes in the education and treatment of patients while assisting a medical doctor. RNs help communicate between the doctor and patient, maintain medical records, and provide instruction. RNs complete either a bachelor's or associate's degree in nursing and do not have the authority to practice independently of a doctor.

NURSE PRACTITIONER (NP)— an RN with advanced training. In addition to the requirements to become an RN, NPs obtain a graduate degree or higher and frequently need work experience as an RN before being accepted into the degree program. In more than 25 states, NPs are able to practice independently from a doctor and can diagnose, treat, and prescribe medication in addition to the duties an RN would perform.

REGISTERED DIETICIAN (RD)— those who are trained to use diet and nutrition to treat disease. They complete a bachelor of science (BS) or master's (MS) degree in dietetics and an internship and pass an exam to receive their credentials. They can work independently or

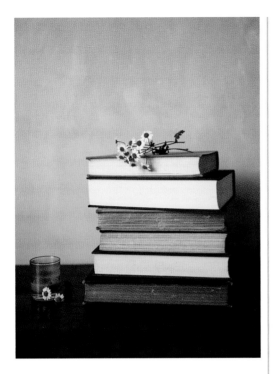

consult with patients as a part of a larger medical practice.

OTHER MEDICAL SPECIALTIES—If your condition affects the teeth, gums, or eyes, you might also consider seeing a **DENTIST (DDS)** or an **OPTOMETRIST (OD)**, who are medical practitioners specializing in these areas. Similarly, a **PHYSICAL THERAPIST (PT OR DPT)** may be needed if you require physical rehabilitation or therapy.

Types of Licensed Natural Medical Practitioners

These are practitioners who go through rigorous training to obtain licensing and certification but are not a part of the conventional medicine system. It is important to note that in some states and with some insurance plans, NDs can be primary care doctors, as well as prescribe many medications and function as the key player on your health-care team (more about that later in this chapter).

NATUROPATHIC DOCTOR (ND)—a medical professional who has obtained a license to diagnose and treat medical conditions by completing naturopathic medical school (generally 4 years after completing a bachelor's degree) and passing a board exam. NDs are educated in the same foundations as a medical doctor, but instead of moving on to specific areas of study, they also learn about natural-healing modalities. An ND employs these natural-healing methods as well as nutrition and lifestyle changes in his or her practice, and in some states is licensed to prescribe conventional prescription medications.

DOCTOR OF CHIROPRACTIC (DC)—a health-care professional who focuses on the disorders of the musculoskeletal and nervous systems. Training consists of chiropractic school (generally 4 years after completing a bachelor's degree) and passing a licensing exam. DCs' doctorate certification is non-medical, and they are not able to prescribe medication like a medical doctor would. Since the nervous system is so integral to whole-body wellness, a lot of chiropractors offer comprehensive diet and lifestyle consulting in addition to adjustments and physical manipulation.

LICENSED ACUPUNCTURIST (LAC)–a natural-health professional who has been trained in Chinese herbology and acupuncture, a treatment that aims to identify and redirect energetic imbalances within the body. Those who have obtained their LAc certification have completed a master's-level program usually encompassing 3 to 4 years after a bachelor's degree. In some states, like California, an LAc can order lab testing, although they are unable to prescribe conventional medications and instead use herbal preparations.

DOCTOR OF ACUPUNCTURE AND ORIENTAL MEDICINE (DOM)–A natural-health professional who has received advanced training (usually 2 years past master's level) in Chinese herbology and acupuncture, with specialties such as gynecology, pain management, and cancer treatment available.

Types of Licensed Complementary Care Practitioners

These are practitioners who go through specific training to provide services that are complementary to conventional medicine. Licenses and certifications can vary by state and by program, so make sure to research to see what kind of training your practitioner has received as well as the types of therapy he or she is licensed to provide.

MASSAGE THERAPIST–a complementary care practitioner who specializes in the physical manipulation of muscles in order to reduce pain, promote relaxation, and ease tension. Massage therapists are required to be trained by an accredited institution and perform massage for a certain number of hours before obtaining certification. Some continue their education and training and become board certified.

COUNSELOR–a practitioner who specializes in helping their clients tackle emotional problems, usually by using talk therapy. Some counselors specialize in certain areas, like addictions, family, marriage, and wellness. Depending on the specialty, counselors obtain a bachelor's degree and/or a master's degree and need to meet practice requirements to obtain licensure and/or board certification.

Types of Nonmedical, Nonlicensed Practitioners

Some complementary therapies face issues such as unlicensed practitioners, not fully backed by scientific research and without acceptance from the medical community, but anecdotally, they have played a role in wellness for many with autoimmune disease. Before delving into this category of treatment options, it is important to have your medical team in place, as your primary need is to receive instruction or treatment from a doctor. We've included a list of some of the more common alternative therapies starting below.

NUTRITION OR HEALTH COACH–a complementary care practitioner who specializes in coaching and advising on a healthy diet. There are a wide variety of certifications, some accredited and some not, and it is possible for a practitioner to become board certified. Nutrition and health coaches who have not completed RD training are not considered medical practitioners and cannot diagnose or treat health conditions.

LIFESTYLE COACH—These practitioners can help you meet a personal goal in a certain area, like wellness. This can be helpful for those who are looking for guidance, recommendations, and encouragement on their journeys. Although there are training programs, the profession is without accreditation or licensing.

HOMEOPATH—These practitioners use the idea that a very small amount of a substance that is known to cause symptoms can actually be used as an agent to relieve those symptoms—the concept of "like cures like." Homeopathic preparations are administered sublingually or by mouth in a dropper.

AYURVEDIC PRACTITIONER—These practitioners employ one of the world's oldest health practices, originating in India, and use foundational concepts about wellness to manage health. Ayurveda calls for dietary changes as well as herbal products as treatment.

REFLEXOLOGIST—a massage therapist who believes that massaging certain points on the feet that are thought to correspond to organs in the body can effect change in the body.

BIOFEEDBACK TECHNICIAN—a practitioner who uses a therapy connecting the body to electrical sensors that monitor impulses, such as heart rate or brain activity. Biofeedback can help you monitor and make changes to your body in real time like relax muscles or reach a meditative state.

MOVEMENT THERAPIST—a teacher of a mind-body practice that involves the therapeutic use of movement or dance to produce desirable changes in the body, either physically or emotionally.

HERBALIST—a practitioner who uses plants for medicinal purposes. Herbalism has deep roots in alternative medicine. Many licensed practitioners (like an ND, LAc, or DOM) as well as many unlicensed practitioners, use herbs in their practices.

REIKI MASSAGE THERAPIST—those who use a Japanese energetic healing modality that involves the placement of hands around the body and balancing energy focusing on body areas in a similar way that an acupuncturist would.

YOGA TEACHER—a teacher who uses a physical practice that can have spiritual and mental components, depending on how it is used, and which involves breathwork and stretching the body. Yoga is practiced in many different styles and as part of many philosophies around the world.

MEDITATION TEACHER—a teacher who uses a practice that aims to benefit the mind by training it to become more present and aware. There are many forms of meditation and ways of achieving this awareness, and some are connected to a spiritual practice, although meditation

The Autoimmune Wellness Handbook

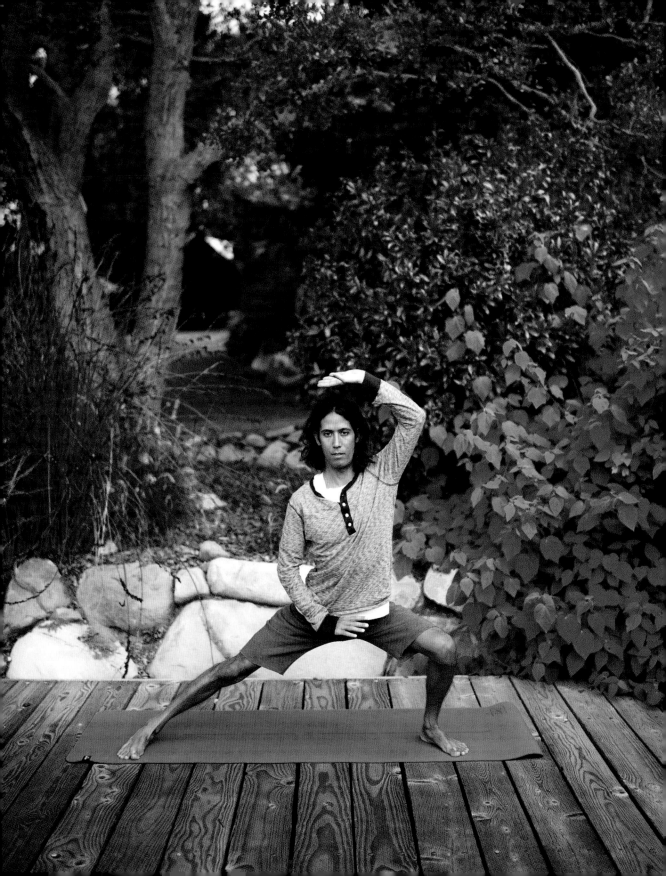

does not need to incorporate spirituality by definition.

Navigating Natural Health-Care Options

Have you found yourself confused at the meaning of some of the words used to describe natural health-care options—*alternative, complementary, integrative,* or *holistic*? Although these words are used to describe treatments in relationship to conventional medicine, their definitions have subtle differences. Before you start to compile your team, it is important to have a working understanding of their meanings.

ANGIE'S EXPERIENCE

Endometriosis is one of the diseases on the list that is only suspected as autoimmune at this time. Medical researchers are still trying to understand the exact nature of the disease. For me, that makes managing my endometriosis with an integrated approach of both natural and conventional medicine an obvious choice. The only way to confirm endometriosis is through a form of surgery called laparoscopy, and currently, the gold-standard treatment is through a technique called excision, performed by extremely skilled surgeons who specialize in treating endometriosis. I have sought out the most skilled surgeons to help me avoid complications. In addition, I use diet, lifestyle, and targeted supplementation based on the advice of my naturopathic doctor to help me best manage the high level of pain that comes with the disease, as well as the hormonal fluctuations that can exacerbate the symptoms.

Know that these terms are neither regulated nor do they signify specific training or certification, although doctors or other health-care practitioners may have received advanced training in these areas. Many providers use these terms to describe their practices or services. It is important to know that it is still up to you to investigate what their interpretation of a complementary approach is, as it can vary widely from practitioner to practitioner.

ALTERNATIVE MEDICINE—when a nonconventional (alternative) treatment is used instead of a conventional one.

COMPLEMENTARY MEDICINE—when nonconventional and conventional treatments are used in conjunction.

INTEGRATIVE MEDICINE—similar to complementary medicine but executed in a coordinated way.

HOLISTIC MEDICINE—when a healing modality addresses the whole person, physically, mentally, and spiritually, instead of that person's parts.

FUNCTIONAL MEDICINE—Like holistic medicine, functional medicine addresses the whole person and aims to uncover the root causes of chronic illness. Practitioners employ diagnostic lab testing and both conventional and natural treatments for both body and mind to produce wellness.

How and When to Integrate a Conventional and Natural Approach

Your decision to use natural therapies in conjunction with or instead of conventional medicine is a personal one. There is no right or wrong way—the path that produces the best health with limited undesirable side effects is your goal. Some people are able to reverse their illnesses merely by using dietary and lifestyle interventions. Others recover using a complementary or integrative approach, using both conventional and natural medical methods. Some have needs that are very deeply rooted in the conventional medical system, making medication or surgery necessary. Your path is unique, and your decision to use natural therapies is dependent on your needs and personal preferences about health care.

Integration of a conventional and natural approach can take many forms. It might look like hiring an integrative MD as your key player (more on that on page 37) and having her guide your care for both general health and autoimmune disease. Or, you may decide to see a conventionally rooted specialist in conjunction with a natural practitioner, such as a gastroenterologist and an ND for the treatment of a digestive disease (like Crohn's or celiac disease). You could choose to see a conventional MD for general health care and employ complementary health-care modalities like chiropractic, massage, and health coaching to fill the gaps. As effective and helpful as natural therapies can be, everyone needs to have a licensed medical practitioner on the team to serve as his or her primary care provider, to perform annual exams, and to be a point of contact for health support.

The integration of a natural approach

has the best chance of success if an illness is caught in the early stages and has not progressed significantly. Many try a natural or complementary approach first, before jumping into more conventional treatments like medication or surgery, especially if those treatments come with undesirable side effects. The flip side is also true—if your illness is severe, you may not have the choice of trying a completely natural approach. Make sure to make this decision with a practitioner who is licensed to advise you on the issue. For instance, don't ask your massage therapist if he can help you avoid surgery!

HOW DO YOU BUILD A COLLABORATIVE TEAM?

Now that you understand what collaboration is, the difference between natural and conventional medicine, the various types of providers, and when to integrate your approach, we need to start talking about exactly how to build a collaborative team.

First, it is important to understand a few key concepts on collaboration.

● **KNOW WHAT IS AT STAKE**—Knowing what you want and how that relates to what those on your team want will help guide your interactions.

● **VALUE DIVERSITY AND DIFFERING OPINIONS**—Instead of expecting every health-care practitioner to have the same opinion about something, value the instances when they all bring something different to the table.

- **LEARN HOW TO HANDLE CONFLICT**—Your health-care team may present you with options that you are not expecting, that you don't agree with, or that conflict with each other. Being patient and handling these situations objectively can help you preserve the integrity of a collaborative relationship.

- **RECOGNIZE THAT COLLABORATION IS A DEVELOPMENTAL PROCESS**—The more you practice collaboration with your health-care team, the easier it will be to continue this style of working relationship as trust builds over time.

- **BALANCE AUTONOMY AND UNITY**—Realize when it is appropriate for you to question your practitioner's plan, when to come together to devise a more unified one, or when to surrender and trust your team. This is a difficult concept and takes experience and practice to develop.

- **RECOGNIZE WHEN COLLABORATION IS NOT NEEDED**—Note when it is appropriate not to collaborate, such as when a problem is not so complex it warrants a whole team to solve it. Sometimes independent decision making by you or particular members of your team is appropriate, especially if involving all voices will make a simple issue complicated.

What does this look like? Collaboration is likely to start with your communicating to your health-care providers about the steps you are taking with other providers or making all parties aware of the offerings of

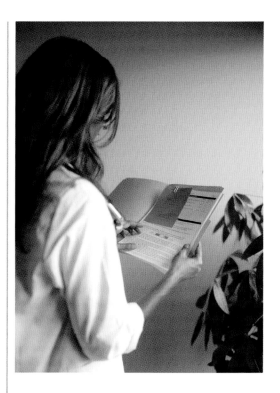

one provider that complement the advice of another. The onus is on you, as the patient, as clear coordination between providers is unfortunately not yet standard practice outside of an extreme health crisis (like a car accident resulting in critical injuries that require multiple medical disciplines to help the patient recover). If you are lucky enough to find providers open and willing to take the time to speak with each other, be sure to support coordination of their efforts.

Next, with those concepts in mind, following is a list of the various roles you need to fill on your team.

- **MVP**—The "most valuable player" on your collaborative health-care team is *you*. It takes time and effort to be part of your team, but an engaged, empowered patient can make or break a quality health-care experience. As the MVP, you need to choose providers wisely, partner with them to determine the best choices for you, understand and communicate what quality care looks like for you, prepare questions to ask and give providers all the information (even the uncomfortable stuff!) they need to do their jobs, come to appointments with your visit goals prioritized, be ready to follow through on recommendations, and be willing to look for new providers if a relationship is not working.

- **KEY PLAYER**—This is the provider who you see first for your needs. It may be an MD or DO who practices primary care medicine or it may be a specialist. This person might also be a PA, NP, or ND. She is your main point of contact and helps provide much of the information and/or direction that the rest of the team needs. Details about choosing your key player can be found in the next column.

- **SUPPORT PLAYERS**—These are all the various support roles required to round out your team. These players could include only one other person or several, depending on your current needs, and cover everyone from crucial family members or friends to other medical doctors, licensed natural medicine practitioners, complementary care practitioners, or nonmedical providers. Details about filling in the supporting roles can be found on page 41.

HOW DO YOU CHOOSE YOUR KEY PLAYER?

Choosing your key player wisely is crucial to building your collaborative health-care team. This provider is going to act as your medical "home." He will be the provider you visit for most health-care needs, from routine screenings for your autoimmune disease to low-level illnesses like a sore throat or stomach bug, to wellness visits where you share extremely private concerns and ask important questions. Ideally, this relationship will last years, even decades, and be the cornerstone of maintaining your good health.

At the very least, all members of your team, but especially your key player, should be respectful, willing collaborators, and great listeners. You should also expect a minimum of clinical care (this means following an established process in meeting your needs), timeliness, and follow-through. This means that your provider is communicating test results and getting you referrals on a timely basis.

With those basics outlined, there are some other significant questions to ask yourself while choosing your key player.

- **WHAT IS MY KEY PLAYER'S BACKGROUND AND EXPERIENCE?** Think about the educational background that is important to you, as well as your provider's experience, especially in caring for someone with your autoimmune disease. That said, don't dismiss younger providers. There is value to both those with more recent training and older providers with years of hands-on practice.

- **IS MY KEY PLAYER "IN-NETWORK" WITH MY INSURANCE PLAN?** Insurance companies have special, discounted rates with certain doctors and hospitals, and using providers and facilities within that rate plan is much less expensive for you. You can check with your insurance plan to find out which doctors are "in-network."

- **DOES MY KEY PLAYER HAVE THE EXPERTISE I NEED OR WANT IN A PROVIDER?** Considering the list of practitioner types starting on page 28, narrow down your choices to a provider who best matches your preferences. In some states, NDs are allowed the same scope of practice as MDs or DOs and you may prefer them as your primary care provider. These scopes of practice do vary widely though, so in thinking about this, be sure that if your autoimmune disease requires medication, an ND will be allowed to prescribe it.

- **DOES ANYONE I KNOW HAVE A GOOD RECOMMENDATION FOR MY KEY PLAYER?** There is no better referral to a provider than those offered by family or friends. Having feedback about an in-person interaction with a potential candidate is invaluable to your decision-making process.

EVALUATING POTENTIAL PROVIDERS CHECKLIST

Here are some questions to ask your potential providers when you schedule the initial visit. Often, their receptionist will be able to answer most of these for you, and if you heard of their practice by referral, other patients may be able to tell you more about their experiences. We have found it best to ask some of these questions before the first appointment to be sure you are not wasting time with a practitioner who does not have the expertise you are looking for or a collaborative spirit.

- ☐ What kind of insurance do they take?
- ☐ How much do their services cost?
- ☐ If you don't have insurance, do they have a "cash price" or a discount?
- ☐ Do they only offer services as part of a package or do they charge by the session?
- ☐ Are they familiar with your condition(s)?
- ☐ Do they have experience or expertise troubleshooting tough cases or working with those who suffer from chronic conditions?
- ☐ How much time do they spend with a patient during an appointment?

- ☐ What is their intake process?
- ☐ Can they be contacted for troubleshooting or follow-up?
- ☐ How busy is their schedule—can you get in to see them on short notice?
- ☐ What is their education/training background?
- ☐ How do they collaborate with other practitioners?
- ☐ Do they require you to purchase supplements from their office?

EVALUATING YOUR CURRENT PROVIDERS CHECKLIST

Here is a list of questions you can use to evaluate the team you have already put in place or the new providers you are considering. Keep in mind that not all providers are going to score high in all areas, but asking yourself these questions will help you determine their weak spots and if you would be better served working with someone else.

- ☐ How caring is their bedside manner?
- ☐ How thorough is their annual physical?
- ☐ Do they practice or are they familiar with natural or alternative approaches?
- ☐ Do they take the time to answer all of your questions?
- ☐ Are they available for troubleshooting or follow-up?
- ☐ Are they familiar with a real food diet and are they happy to support it?
- ☐ Are they familiar with your autoimmune disease?
- ☐ Are they willing to discuss and order, when necessary, testing that you want done?
- ☐ Are they willing to discuss and refer you, when necessary, to specialists you want to see?
- ☐ Are they open-minded about using natural methods before prescribing pharmaceuticals?
- ☐ Are they cautious when recommending medications and supplements or do they tend to be heavy-handed?
- ☐ Do they seem concerned with your long-term well-being and progress?
- ☐ Are they collaborative—are they including you and other team members in decision making?

- **DO I WANT MY KEY PLAYER CLOSE TO MY HOME OR WORK?** Maybe choosing a provider who is located close to your office makes a lot more sense than one close to your home. Perhaps traveling a relatively long distance for a very worthwhile provider is something you are willing to do. Consider location in your decision.

- **HOW ACCESSIBLE IS MY KEY PLAYER?** You should be able to get in to see your provider within reasonable time frames. If you can't actually see the provider, you won't be able to get the help you need. If sick visits, for instance, cannot be scheduled within 24 hours, that might be a sign that the fit is not good. On the other hand, needing to schedule a well visit several weeks to a month out is usually acceptable.

- **DOES MY KEY PLAYER AND HER STAFF PRACTICE GOOD RECORD KEEPING?** Your provider will not be able to offer much help if she is not properly noting, tracking, and storing your health data. Along with this, consider whether or not she uses electronic records, which can make communication with your other team members quite a bit easier and allow you to access your own information more smoothly.

- **IS THE CUSTOMER SERVICE OF MY KEY PLAYER'S STAFF UP TO PAR?** If you find yourself getting nervous about the likely negative encounter you will have each time you have to contact the office, that is a red flag. You will have to "pass the gate" every time you interact with your doctor, and you don't want to be consistently treated poorly or with lack of concern.

Once you've chosen your key player, it's time to schedule a first visit and use that initial encounter to assess if she is able to fulfill this role on your team. On page 38, you'll see a list of questions to ask when

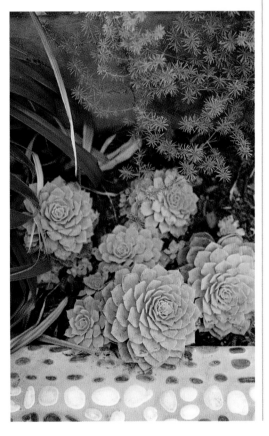

you schedule that initial visit. If she turns out to be right for you, following that meeting, you can move on to filling the supporting roles on your health-care team. Otherwise, you should continue your search for your key player before getting any further along in building your team.

How Do You Fill the Support Player Roles?

Making careful choices for the support players on your health-care team isn't quite as critical to a quality health-care experience as choosing your key player, but they are still important. Great support can make your journey a true success, while poor matches can make wellness goals nearly impossible to achieve. The kinds of people filling your support roles are more varied than those in the key player position and your need for them can change a lot depending on where you are with your disease. For instance, these players could be a vital family member or friend acting as your advocate and/or caretaker; various medical specialists relevant to your diagnosis; complementary care practitioners like a chiropractor, acupuncturist, or therapist, whom you only need for a relatively short period of time; or nonmedical providers like a health coach or yoga teacher who will help you achieve very specific goals.

The support roles are the last pieces to round out your team and make your healing a holistic (whole-body) process. Your key player cannot be expected to know everything and be everything at all times for you. Try as she might, it is rare for only one provider to be capable of meeting all of your needs, yet healing as a whole person is a valuable goal. For this reason, striving to fill support roles on your team is worth all the effort. A very basic and typical support team might include a disease specialist (if your key player is not a specialist to begin with), a counselor, and a family member or friend.

Again, at the very least, your support providers should be respectful, willing collaborators, and great listeners. You should also expect a minimum of clinical care (where appropriate—this obviously does not apply in the case of family or friends), timeliness, and follow-through.

With those basics outlined, here are some other things to consider while choosing your support players.

● **WHAT HELP WOULD MOST BENEFIT YOU IN ADDITION TO YOUR KEY PLAYER?** Determine all the additional supports, perhaps along with your key player's recommendations, that would best meet your needs. Once your ideal list is in place, begin considering your time availability and financial resources in order to trim the team to what is most practical for you.

● **DO YOU NEED A MEDICAL SPECIALIST OR SPECIALISTS FOR YOUR AUTOIMMUNE DIAGNOSIS(ES)?** If so, are there providers "in-network" with your insurance plan? Your key player may recommend one or you may

want a specialist to help you dig deeper. For instance, a gastroenterologist if you have celiac disease or a dermatologist if you have psoriasis can be invaluable.

● **DO YOU NEED ANY LICENSED COMPLEMENTARY CARE PROVIDERS?** If so, will your insurance plan cover all or a portion of their services? Some plans cover acupuncture, chiropractic care, massage, physical therapy, or counseling. Be sure to check and take advantage of coverage if it is offered.

● **WILL YOU NEED TO SEE YOUR SUPPORT PLAYER OFTEN?** If so, a convenient location may be important. Support players frequently offer routine care that needs to happen on a regular, ongoing basis, such as weekly massage or talk therapy sessions.

● **DO YOU HAVE ONE CLOSE FAMILY MEMBER OR FRIEND WHOM YOU CAN LEAN ON?** What you need from this person can be considerable when you are still very debilitated but much less when you are enjoying greater health. Be sensitive to the fact that your needs may be too large a burden or this person may not be able to support you in all the ways you require. If that is the case, express your gratitude for what she is able to give and then add a second, third, or fourth family member or friend to your team. For example, maybe your partner is able to do extra chores and go to appointments with you, but not able to listen when you need to vent about your illness. Finding a friend to vent to, particularly someone who has a similar diagnosis, fills that need and also relieves some of the pressure from your partner. The more robust your network, the better!

In addition to these considerations, you may also want to ask yourself some of the same questions you did while choosing your key player. Once you've chosen your support players, schedule first visits and treat those sessions as interviews. In the case of that vital family member or friend, schedule a time to talk with her that is best for both of you and without distractions. Be open and frank about your needs and express how much it would mean to you to have her love and support as you seek healing. Graciously asking for help, rather than taking it for granted, is likely to win you a devoted partner for the path ahead.

Conflicting Advice

If you are deciding to use both conventional and complementary care health-care providers, it is inevitable that you will face the issue of conflicting advice, opinions, or treatment options. This can happen even if you're just using one mode or the other. This is a frustrating experience that can lead you to lose trust in your health-care team.

Here are some tips for managing conflicting advice.

- **DO EVERYTHING YOU CAN TO PRESERVE COLLABORATION ON YOUR TEAM.** Be patient, open, and honest with your practitioners. Let them know who else is on your team and be clear about when conflicts arise so they can help be a part of the solution.

- **ALWAYS VALUE THE ADVICE OF YOUR KEY PLAYER OVER ALL OTHER PRACTITIONERS.** This is one of the most important reasons why having a collaborative, experienced, and supportive doctor as your key player is absolutely necessary. If your key player is not up to par, you may be faced with lack of trust and confusion about his recommendations and how they relate to others on your health-care team.

- **BE SUSPECT OF MEDICAL ADVICE FROM NONMEDICAL PRACTITIONERS.** While it is true that a lot of natural therapies can help medical conditions, it is not the place of nonlicensed or nonmedical practitioners to make claims or prescribe the treatment of disease. If a nonmedical practitioner is trying to give you advice that affects your medication or treatment, make sure to run it by your doctor or licensed medical practitioner, and heed his opinion above that of any complementary care practitioners.

- **GET A SECOND OPINION.** Especially in the face of serious medications and/or surgery, don't forget that you can always see another practitioner for her take on it.

- **ALWAYS RESPECT YOUR INSTINCTS.** In the end, it is your choice, not your doctor's or anyone else's on your health-care team, what you do regarding your own body. If a piece of advice continues not to sit well with your own inner guidance system, take it as a sign that you need to do more research and possibly consult another person before moving forward with it.

Should You Ever Fire a Provider?

It can be stressful changing health-care providers. People often find the process of leaving a provider, even if they know it is not a good match, so daunting that they stay in bad working relationships. While we understand how hard it can be to find someone new, we encourage you to move on if there are signs that your current provider is not working out. This is particularly true with your key player. The members of your health-care team are there to help you, so making sure these links are as strong as possible matters.

The following are some red flags that it's time to say goodbye.

- **NEED AND STYLE MISMATCH**—Some patients prefer very blunt, direct providers; others prefer lots of empathy. Some patients like a formal provider, while others like a relaxed approach. If what you prefer isn't the style of your provider, you may not mesh in the long term.

- **LACK OF CONTINUITY**—If there is no follow-through on your provider's part between visits, or every time you return for an appointment, your provider seems to be encountering your history for the very first time, this is a bad sign. A connection

should form and consistent care should be happening between visits.

- **NEED-TO-KNOW BASIS**—If your provider keeps you in the dark about the reason behind tests, treatments, or even certain results, it is time to go. It is your right to know why he wants to take specific steps, and a lack of openness or inability to speak with you about it in a straightforward manner (without complicated medical jargon) is a bad sign. In the same vein, if you don't feel comfortable giving your provider *all* of the detail he needs about your health, and you are essentially keeping him in the dark, this is also a bad sign.

- **DISMISSIVE ATTITUDE**—A provider should welcome your questions and concerns, willingly addressing them. She should also listen carefully to what you have learned, as well as your noted symptoms and instincts on what is happening in your body. It is a significant problem if you repeatedly see your provider about a concerning issue and she repeatedly disregards it or makes assumptions without paying attention to what you've said.

- **LACK OF RESPECT**—You are the authority on your body, hands down. If the provider is plainly rude, condescending, or disrespectful, you should definitely fire him.

- **UNWILLING COLLABORATOR**—Your provider should be ready to coordinate with the other members of your team, take into account any new information they have provided, and talk with you about the instructions and recommendations they are giving you. If he views himself as a "one-man show," that can be a sign that the working relationship is not going to be productive.

- **UNAVAILABILITY**—Being able to get in touch with your provider between appointments for any follow-up questions or to report any concerns with medications or treatments is important. If she is unreachable, that's a sign that your partnership is unlikely to work out.

- **ALWAYS BEING KEPT WAITING**—Sometimes, having a provider who is consistently a bit late for your appointment is actually a good sign. He may be very thorough and dedicated, taking ample time with each patient, including you. However, if you are constantly sitting in a cold exam room as the minutes (or worse yet, hours!) tick away, this shows how much the provider undervalues your time. This also applies to get-

ting in for appointments. If you have to wait for months at a time to get in, the practice may be too busy to realistically meet your individual needs.

If you decide to fire your provider, it does not need to be a dramatic confrontation. Simply write a letter stating your reasons for leaving and requesting your medical records. Making sure you have the best possible players on your health-care team is absolutely worth the effort.

THE BIG DECISIONS

Medication and Surgery

You may have started your research about alternative therapies after your medical doctor advised medication and/or surgery. There are many reasons why you wouldn't want to take these approaches, considering the potential side effects, invasiveness, and permanence that come with some treatments. You could also already be on a laundry list of medications, experiencing various side effects, and wishing to do away with them. Before taking action, however, make sure to read this section carefully as it is a tricky and personal subject.

As we mentioned in Chapter 1, the conventional treatment for managing some autoimmune diseases can involve pharmaceutical medications and surgery. As an alternative or complement to this approach, integrative and functional medicine practitioners have additional tools in their toolbox, sometimes being able to minimize or avoid these drastic measures. In addition, the changes you can make for yourself to your diet and lifestyle may have an impact on your need for medication or surgery. After employing these approaches, you may find that you can avoid conventional treatment like surgery or are able to wean off your medications, in collaboration with your doctor.

Does Needing Medication or Surgery Mean You've Failed?

Sometimes it is clear to you and your medical team that medication and/or surgery is the only choice. When faced with this situation, especially after trying to implement some complementary therapies, you may assume that you've failed entirely—this could not be further from the truth! Instead, your goal should be living to your highest standard of wellness with autoimmune disease. Although we advocate for a complementary approach to medical care as well as dietary and lifestyle changes, we never suggest avoiding necessary medication and/or surgery.

Here are some common instances where medication and/or surgery may be necessary.

- **YOU LACK AN IMPORTANT HORMONE FOR OPTIMAL FUNCTION.** This is common in autoimmune diseases like type 1 diabetes or Hashimoto's thyroiditis, where tissue destruction prevents the body from making hormones that are crucial for optimal health (in this case, insulin or thyroid hormone).

- **YOUR SYMPTOMS ARE DEBILITATING.** Some autoimmune diseases cause symptoms that render a person unable to function in daily life, whether that is inflammation, pain, or something else. There are medications that can make this more manageable, such as those that relieve pain for rheumatoid arthritis.

- **YOU HAVE SIGNIFICANT TISSUE DAMAGE.** In the case of inflammatory bowel disease (Crohn's disease and ulcerative colitis), sometimes tissue damage is so widespread that surgery is necessary for repair and optimal function. In the case of endometriosis, growths may need to be removed in order to preserve organ function.

Many of us who suffer from autoimmune disease have employed pharmaceutical or surgical treatments at key or ongoing points in our healing journeys, in conjunction with natural treatments, and credit them for our recovery and ongoing health. Mickey takes replacement thyroid hormone to control her Hashimoto's thyroiditis, and Angie has undergone laparoscopic surgery to manage her endometriosis. There is no reason to feel like a failure if you are doing everything in your power to educate yourself and effectively manage your condition.

Can You Wean Off Your Medications?

It is absolutely possible for you to wean off some, if not all, medications using a natural approach, but it is important to note that this may not be an outcome for everyone—it depends on your current condition and disease progression. *This is something that needs to be handled under the care and supervision of your medical team and never on your own.*

If weaning off medications is your goal, the first step is to have a clear conversation with your medical practitioner, letting her know about any complementary approaches you may be employing that she is not aware of (including dietary and lifestyle changes) and asking for her help with the possibility of more frequent monitoring and weaning, if she decides it is medically possible. Espe-

cially with the implementation of dietary and lifestyle modifications, it is more likely that you will experience changes in areas like blood pressure, cholesterol, blood sugar, reflux, and constipation before experiencing changes in your more serious autoimmune symptoms. Thus, weaning off medications can be a long-term process that goes in phases as you restore your health.

How Do You Stretch Your Health-Care Dollars?

The unbelievable price of health care, particularly in the United States, sometimes makes it difficult to justify the idea that your health is more valuable than anything else. Although most of us with autoimmune diseases know, instinctively and from experience, that without good health, nothing else matters, it can still be unpleasant receiving sizable medical bills. We did not think this chapter would be complete without some practical suggestions on deciding when and where to spend and when to pull back.

- **ADJUST YOUR LIFESTYLE FOR THE GREATEST AMOUNT OF SELF-CARE.** This should go without saying and the rest of this book will explain exactly how, but you need to change your life to give yourself the best possible chances for optimal health. Dedicate the bulk of your health-care budget to maximize self-care—things like eating well and taking advantage of that gym membership! We will be talking more about this in Chapter 5.

- **UNDERSTAND YOUR INSURANCE PLAN BENEFITS AND PAY CLOSE ATTENTION.** Educate

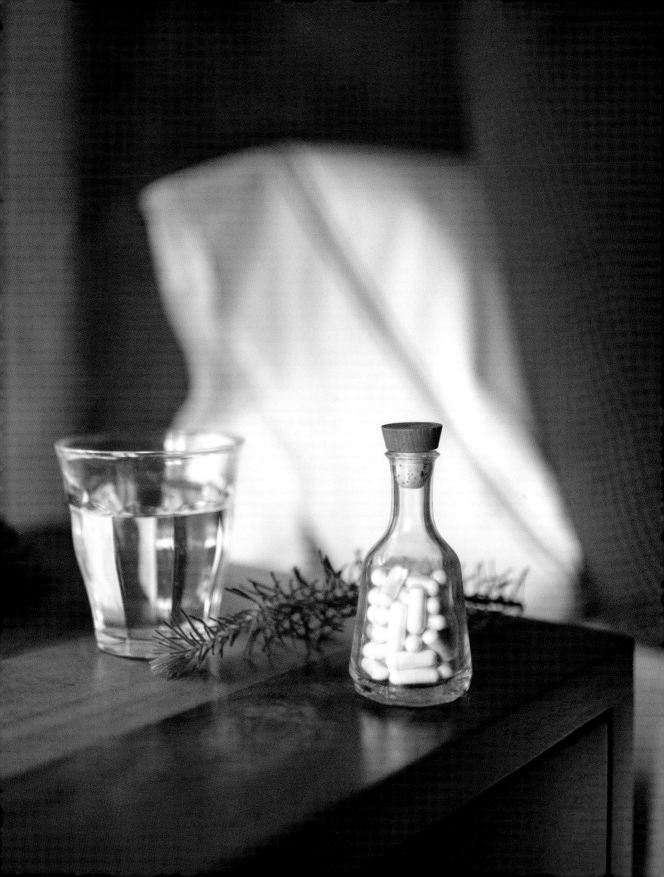

yourself on the finer points of what is covered, what is not covered, the coverage approval process, and, as discussed earlier, the doctors and hospitals that are "in-network." Then be prepared to follow up closely. If you feel your insurance company has denied payment incorrectly or has not paid what they are obligated to pay, dedicate time and effort to getting your full benefit. You may also need to work this same approach with providers and hospitals. This can be extremely stressful and time-consuming work, so finding a partner who can help you stay on top of reviewing bills and seeking maximum benefits is a great idea. You will usually be able to save substantial amounts of money if you are diligent with this process.

● **GET THE MOST THOROUGH ANNUAL EXAM POSSIBLE AND MAKE THE MOST OF THE INFORMATION GAINED.** Preventive care is key. Use your annual exam as your primary information-gathering appointment of the year. You will particularly want to pay close attention to your lab results. Take time to learn about them and discuss the results with your provider. If you see results that are questionable, even if your provider seems to feel they are acceptable, schedule a follow-up to talk about them further. This is your chance to advocate for yourself and potentially identify and correct health problems before they get out of control. In addition, if there are tests that can be routinely done for you to stay on top of your autoimmune disease, learn all you can about those tests and have them conducted at regular intervals.

● **ASK ABOUT PAYMENT PLANS OR CASH PRICING WITH PROVIDERS NOT COVERED BY INSURANCE.** For any members of your health-care team who are not covered by your insurance plan, be sure to ask about payment plan options or if they offer discounted pricing for clients who pay cash. Many of these providers are willing to work with clients on payment for extensive care that may be difficult to pay out-of-pocket.

There are also times when it is important to evaluate whether or not spending makes sense. Occasionally, it might be a good idea to stop spending and pump the health-care brakes.

Here are some suggestions on being more selective.

● **AN EXPENSIVE REPEAT TEST IS BEING SUGGESTED FOR AN ISSUE YOU ARE NOW VERY FAMILIAR WITH.** If you can recognize symptoms of a particular issue yourself, let your provider know and ask if you can avoid testing and proceed based on symptom evaluation. An example of this might be urinary tract infections, which many women recognize without testing.

● **AN EXPENSIVE TEST NOT COVERED BY YOUR INSURANCE IS BEING SUGGESTED AND THE INFORMATION IT WILL PROVIDE IS NOT CRUCIAL TO YOUR HEALTH CARE AT THIS TIME.** For instance, comprehensive stool analysis can provide extremely useful information, but may not be necessary to repeat frequently. Ask your provider if holding off in order to save money is appropriate.

- **A VERY INVASIVE TEST IS BEING SUGGESTED AND THE INFORMATION IT WILL PROVIDE IS NOT CRUCIAL TO YOUR HEALTH CARE AT THIS TIME.** Perhaps your provider is proposing your third endoscopy in the last 2 years and you just don't feel capable of going through the procedure again or are worried about the expense. Express your concerns and work with him to decide if it is truly worthwhile or if it can wait.

- **YOU ARE HAVING A SCARY HEALTH PROBLEM, BUT YOU KNOW FROM EXPERIENCE THAT THE ER IS NOT NECESSARY.** With some autoimmune diseases, upsetting symptoms can sometimes come up, but over time, you may be able to distinguish between a major medical emergency and a scary, but not life-threatening, scenario. If you are in this situation and just need to calm any fears, consider going to an urgent care clinic and getting advice on how to proceed. It is much less expensive, not to mention less stressful, than the ER. (*Naturally, we are not advocating skipping the ER if you need it, only stating that if you understand your health challenges well, you can be more judicious in how to treat them.*)

- **AN EXPENSIVE SUPPLEMENT IS BEING SUGGESTED, BUT YOU CAN POTENTIALLY GET IT FROM A FOOD SOURCE OR WAIT TO ADD IT TO YOUR ROUTINE.** Do your research on any supplements your providers suggest and seek out expert opinions before buying. If you think you might be able to get the nutrients in the supplement from your diet or that it is not essential at this time, ask your provider about holding off on it and re-evaluating its addition to your routine later.

- **AN EXPENSIVE FORM OF COMPLEMENTARY CARE HAS BEEN SUGGESTED, BUT YOU DON'T NOTICE A MAJOR BENEFIT WITHIN 30 TO 60 DAYS.** An example of this might be acupuncture or massage, as for some it may be extremely beneficial, while for others it doesn't seem to have the desired impact. Don't feel you have to carry on with this kind of care if it is not benefiting you. Instead, ask your provider if another form of care would be a better fit or what the reasons for lack of results could be so that you can assess how best to spend your money.

In general, people do not regret money spent on maintaining good health. The cost burden can be very high for those of us dealing with the chronic nature of autoimmune disease, but you never hear anyone say, "I seriously regret investing that money in my health." Nothing else matters if you don't have your health. That is easy to take for granted when you are well, but dramatically obvious when you are unwell. You can't enjoy all the things you could do with the money spent on health care, if you can't leave your bed anyway, right? The enormous expense also forces us to take action and responsibility, to be full participants in our own care. And *that* can be an empowering breakthrough!

PRIORITIZING ACTION FLOWCHART

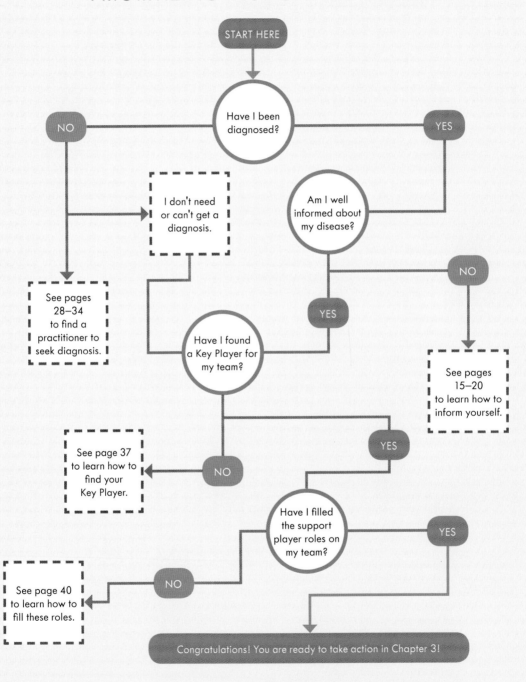

START HERE

Have I been diagnosed?

NO

YES

I don't need or can't get a diagnosis.

Am I well informed about my disease?

NO

See pages 28–34 to find a practitioner to seek diagnosis.

YES

See pages 15–20 to learn how to inform yourself.

Have I found a Key Player for my team?

See page 37 to learn how to find your Key Player.

NO

YES

Have I filled the support player roles on my team?

YES

NO

See page 40 to learn how to fill these roles.

Congratulations! You are ready to take action in Chapter 3!

The Autoimmune Wellness Handbook

CALL TO ACTION

Forming a collaborative health-care team to help manage your care is a substantial undertaking, but it is at the core of the autoimmune wellness journey. Seeking out the help of others, specifically those with necessary expertise, can dramatically change the course of your disease. It is our intention to present a complete picture of what collaboration means and how to put it into practice with your team. Understanding the various approaches to health care, the kinds of practitioners available to assist you, how to choose the players who will come alongside you, and the big treatment and spending decisions they will present you with, allows you to truly be a collaborator in your own care. None of us is an island in this life. It is working together, learning to *collaborate*, that is the best way to achieve any goal.

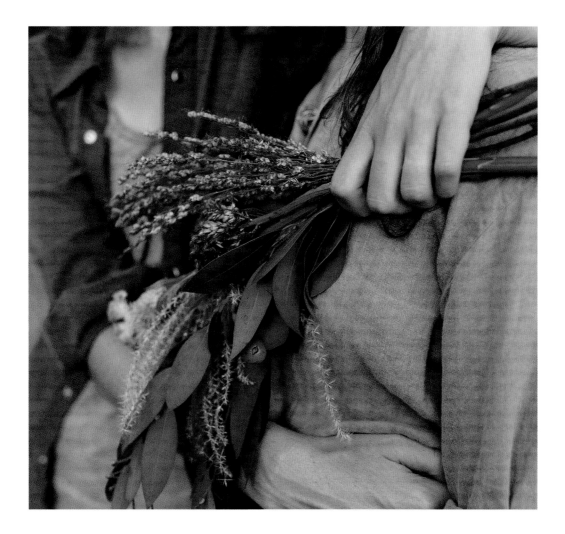

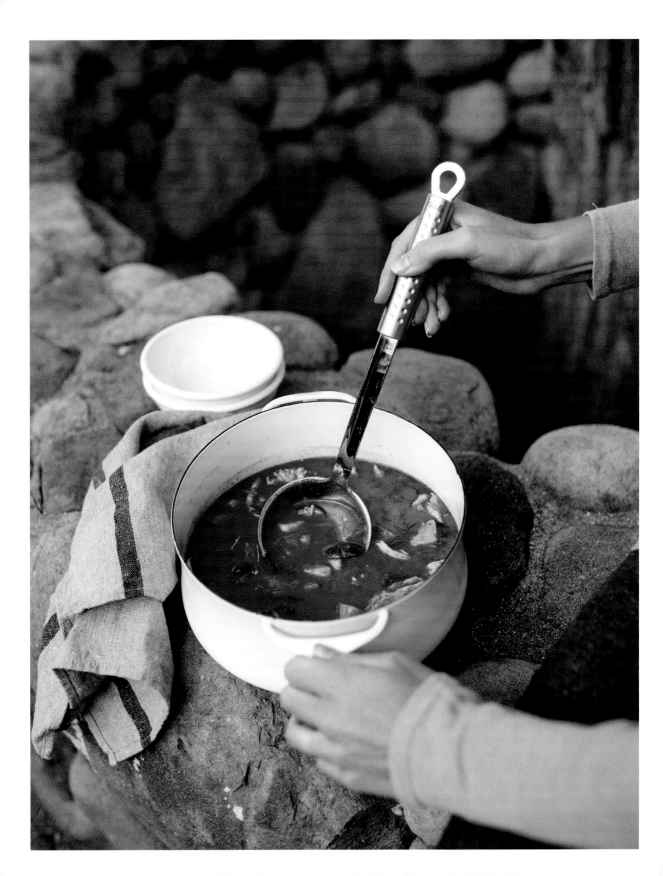

CHAPTER 3

Nourish

"It is not an exaggeration to say that gut health is everything. The health of your gut has a profound effect on your overall health." —Sarah Ballantyne, PhD, *The Paleo Approach*

USING DIETARY MODIFICATIONS TO MANAGE AUTOIMMUNE disease is far from a conventional approach. However, as research continues to clarify the link between what transpires in our guts and how that relates to our immune systems, it is becoming more widely accepted in the medical community. When inquiring with your doctor about the role diet plays in better managing your condition, you may have been told that it has no influence. This could not be further from the truth! We are here to tell you that *what you eat does matter*, and it can have a profound impact on your healing journey. The foods you choose to eat every day provide your body with the raw materials it needs to perform optimally. Whether your diet is a source of nourishment or strain depends on the particular foods you choose to put on your plate.

After informing yourself about your condition and getting your health-care team solidly in place, it is time for you to assess your diet. The cornerstone of living well with autoimmune disease is eating a diet that best supports your long-term health and well-being. This way of eating is going to be unique to you (no one-size-fits-all approach here!). Avoiding foods that you may be allergic or sensitive to, adding more nutrition where you need it, and preventing or controlling imbalances in gut flora can profoundly accelerate and strengthen the healing process. In the same vein, an improper diet can have a hand in causing inflammation and an exacerbation of symptoms. Figuring out what to eat can be one of the most transformative moments in your healing journey, and not one to take lightly!

Let's go over the four key reasons why diet is a powerful component of healing.

● **INTESTINAL PERMEABILITY/LEAKY GUT**— Research has shown that the common thread linking all autoimmune diseases is indeed in the gut, and is known by the terms *leaky gut* or *intestinal permeability.* Simply put, this happens when the lining of your small intestine (the organ responsible for selectively choosing to let nutrients in and keep pathogens out) becomes more permeable (leaky), thereby letting some of the contents pass into your bloodstream or lymphatic system. Your immune system is then left to deal with these undigested proteins, viruses, bacteria, and toxins that shouldn't be there in the first place, causing more inflammation and potentially setting off an immune response. What causes leaky gut in the first place? Food allergies and sensitivities (especially to gluten, a protein found in some grains), dysbiosis (the imbalance of gut flora), medications, and even stress and overexercise can cause the lining of the small intestine to become more permeable. By removing or reducing these triggers, you lower the burden on your immune system, leading to less inflammation and fewer symptoms.

- **NUTRIENT DEFICIENCIES**—Our modern diet is nutrient poor, lacking many essential vitamins, minerals, and other nutrients needed for well-being. Rapidly declining nutrient levels in our soils (making fewer nutrients available in the fruits and vegetables that we eat) as well as widespread digestive dysfunction compound this problem. Nutrient deficiencies are thought to contribute to the development of autoimmune diseases, with deficiencies in some nutrients (like vitamin D) scientifically linked to their development. Deficiencies can also exacer-

bate the symptoms of autoimmune diseases and worsen the inflammatory process. Those who suffer from autoimmune disease have a greater need for nutrients, especially those that are involved in tissue repair and modulating the immune system. In order to have the best chance at managing your condition, you need to make sure digestion is functioning optimally and that you are getting all nutrients needed to heal your body and decrease inflammation.

- **FOOD ALLERGIES, INTOLERANCES, AND SENSITIVITIES**—Eating foods you are allergic, intolerant, or sensitive to can hinder the healing process. While there are differences in the mechanism and severity of how allergies, intolerances, and sensitivities work, getting to the root of which dietary triggers are affecting you can help you get on the road to recovery.

- **DYSBIOSIS**—Our digestive tract is lined with living microorganisms like bacteria and yeasts, with many playing an essential and supportive role (such as digesting food, producing B vitamins and vitamin K, modulating the immune system, and absorbing nutrients). Dysbiosis is a term used to indicate an imbalance in these populations of microorganisms in the gut, whether it is from pathogens (such as a parasite or bacteria that causes disease) or overgrowths of otherwise helpful inhabitants of the gut (such as small intestine bacterial overgrowth, where beneficial bacteria usually found in the large intestine migrate up into the small intestine). Restoring this balance of gut flora can go a long way in helping promote overall health.

In an effort to make this information more manageable, we won't be delving more deeply into the above topics. For further research, we recommend the fantastic resource *The Paleo Approach* by Sarah Ballantyne, PhD. She presents a thorough scientific analysis of each of these dietary factors that contribute to autoimmune disease.

WHY IS THERE NO ONE-SIZE-FITS-ALL APPROACH TO DIET?

Although making dietary changes can have a major impact on your health and recovery, there is no standard formula to eating for those with autoimmune disease. This can be frustrating! It is important to know that what works for someone else's current state of health may not work for your seemingly similar issues. There are crucial foundations that we can all apply to our diets for best success, but not everyone needs to be on an excessively restricted diet for life. Instead, we encourage you to do some experimenting to find the *least-restricted* diet that is *most likely* to produce long-term health.

In the following section, we will present you with a range of healing diets, from what we would consider the least extreme of the dietary approaches (and for healing purposes, the bare minimum intervention) moving along to the most extreme. You can use this list to modify your diet from the top down, gradually working on finding the least-restricted approach that produces

results. Alternatively, you can jump right into an elimination diet like the Autoimmune Protocol.

DIETARY CHOICES
Gluten-Free Diet

Dr. Ballantyne says it best—"Although the exact role that gluten plays in most autoimmune diseases is elusive, the link between gluten sensitivity is so compelling that many experts in the field believe that gluten sensitivity may contribute to all autoimmune diseases." Because of this, we recommend a strict gluten-free diet as the minimum dietary intervention for anyone suffering from an autoimmune or autoimmune-related condition. Although this sounds harsh, the research is clear. Gluten is not something you want to be consuming if you are committed to long-term healing!

A gluten-free diet is one that avoids all foods that contain gluten, a protein found in grains such as wheat, barley, rye, and triticale. According to conventional medicine, a gluten-free diet is only necessary for those with celiac disease; however, there is a growing body of evidence showing that it is possible for nonceliacs to experience a sensitivity to gluten-containing foods (called nonceliac gluten sensitivity). While celiac disease is characterized by a reaction to two parts of the gluten compound (transglutaminase and alpha-gliadin), many other components of wheat and gluten have been identified as potential triggers for those with nonceliac gluten sensitivity.

Remember leaky gut, the common

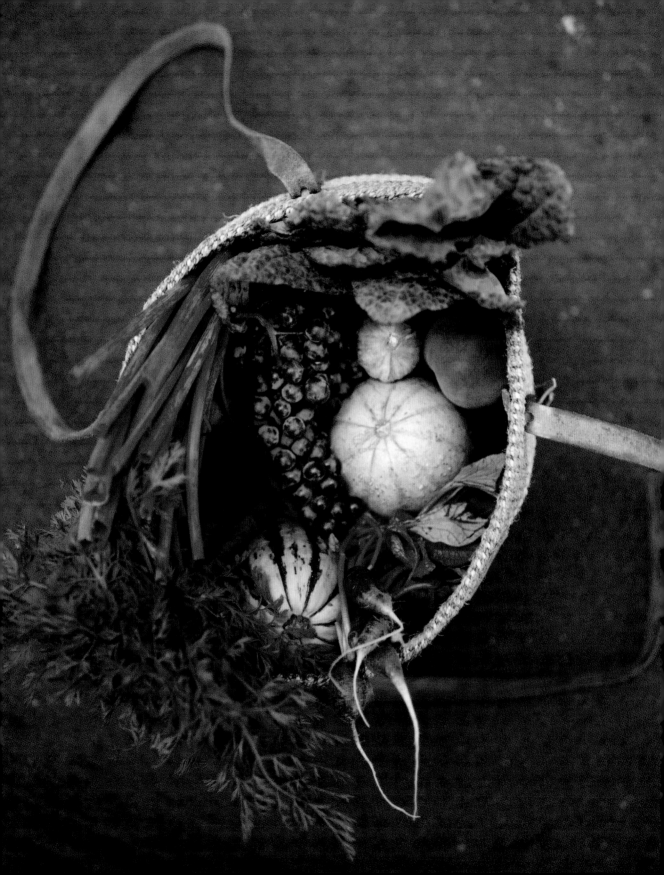

thread linking all autoimmune diseases? Well, it turns out that gluten is exceptionally irritating to the lining of the small intestine, and it has been shown to exacerbate leaky gut and activate the immune system. There is anecdotal evidence that some autoimmune conditions have been put into remission simply by avoiding gluten (and we are not just talking about celiac disease!*). If you are feeling overwhelmed at where to start with dietary intervention, going on a gluten-free diet is a great start.

Dairy-Free Diet

A dairy-free diet is one that avoids all forms of milk products, including but not limited to butter, cheese, milk, yogurt, and all prepared or processed foods containing or made from these ingredients. Although dairy is tolerated by some people, the vast majority, especially those with leaky gut and autoimmune disease, have trouble with it for one reason or another. Depending on your ethnicity, you have a 25 to 97 percent chance of not being able to digest lactose, a sugar found in dairy products. Dairy proteins, in general, are hard to digest and a common food allergy. Even in healthy individuals, dairy products can cause mucous production that worsens symptoms and irritates the gut. Those with a sensitivity to gluten tend to be more sensitive to dairy, as dairy proteins have been shown to cross-react with (mimic) those of gluten. If you

are intolerant to gluten, your body may treat dairy proteins similarly.

Not all dairy is created equal—Some people tolerate some forms and types of dairy better than others (for instance, some may tolerate ghee, butter, and hard cheese but not milk, while others do well with goat but not cow dairy). Because dairy is likely to be a problem for many, we recommend removing it from the diet strictly and then considering reintroducing high-quality dairy slowly once a recovery is made. Some people find their tolerance to dairy changes as they heal their guts, and they may be able to reintroduce high-quality dairy later on in the process, even if they had trouble with it earlier.

Sugar-Free Diet

Excess sugar consumption is a serious issue presented by our modern diet. The low-fat craze has led to the reformulation of processed foods, with the fat being replaced by refined sugar and contributing to the epidemics of obesity and diabetes. Many are becoming mindful of the amount of sugar they consume and seeing results by drastically reducing or cutting it entirely out of their diets.

While sugar specifically does not pose a problem for those with autoimmune disease, excess sugar consumption leads to blood-sugar imbalances, which you may experience as "highs" immediately following consumption and "lows" once your

*If you or anyone on your health-care team suspects that you may have celiac disease, you will want to request antibody testing before you begin a gluten-free diet, as your results may be inaccurate after adopting this way of eating.

blood sugar drops. Over time, this develops into insulin resistance, which means that inflammation has rendered the hormones your body uses to control your blood-sugar levels useless. It is impossible to control inflammation and manage your autoimmune condition unless your blood sugar is under control! Furthermore, excess sugar in the diet can be responsible for feeding pathogenic overgrowths in the gut, exacerbating leaky gut and dysbiosis. Last, sugar weakens the immune system and is a source of empty calories that potentially replace more nutrient-rich foods.

A sugar-free diet can have many variations but, at its simplest, a person avoids all refined sugar and the foods that contain it. While natural sweeteners like honey and maple syrup are considered healthier alternatives by some, their effect on blood sugar is the same—don't be fooled into thinking that there is such a thing as healthy sugar! Sugar substitutes are equally problematic, with many of them being marketed as healthy alternatives despite having a detrimental effect on blood-sugar control, appetite, or containing substances that are known to be toxic.

What about fruit? Although some fruit can have a lot of sugar, in general, fresh, whole fruit is a different story because it contains fiber, vitamins, and minerals in a complete package. While dried fruit should be avoided on a sugar-free diet because of how concentrated and easy to overeat it is, fresh fruit is usually fine to include (and

we'd argue, healthy, because of all of the great nutrients it provides!).

In general, if you aren't already mindful of your sugar consumption, we recommend trying a sugar-free approach for a period of time to better control your blood sugar. Once you cut out sugar, you will become (sometimes painfully!) aware of how dependent your body is on this substance. It is important to take it easy, not cut out too many foods at the same time (like fresh fruit), and make sure you always have healthy protein and fat-rich snacks on hand to navigate those harder moments. Over time, your body will become more dependent on its own stores of energy and your blood sugar will become more stable.

Where do treats fit in? For those who are not experiencing blood-sugar issues, naturally sweetened treats (those with honey, maple syrup, etc.) should be fine occasionally. Fruit should be consumed according to tolerance and preference and not avoided (except for dried varieties, especially in those with more of a sensitivity to sugar). While some forms of sugar, as well as the processed foods in which it lurks, can be incredibly problematic and should be avoided, you should be able to reach a place of balance with sugar consumption that is enjoyable and healthy.

Paleo and Ancestral Diets

The Paleo diet is an approach to eating that has become popular in both the wellness as well as chronic illness communities, with many doctors, researchers, and health experts advocating for its usefulness in combating illness and disease. Paleo is a scientific approach based on the pre-agricultural diet of our ancestors, bypassing all of our modern processed, convenience, and nutrient-poor foods.

Following a Paleo approach, you would avoid grains, beans, legumes, dairy, refined sugar, refined oils, and food chemicals. Ideally, you would also be eating pasture-raised and grass-fed meat and eggs, wild-caught fish, as well as making use of the "odd bits" like bones and organ meats. Paleo also emphasizes fermented foods in order to promote healthy gut flora.

We advocate for adopting a Paleo diet for long-term healing, whether you land there by gradually eliminating foods or by working backward from an elimination diet. Although Paleo can incorporate foods some people are still sensitive to (eggs, nuts, seeds, and the nightshade family of plants), it is generally a nutrient-dense and healthy way of eating because it avoids processed foods and grains that can be problematic for those with autoimmune disease.

Elimination Diet

An elimination diet is a short-term approach where foods are eliminated for a set period of time and then reintroduced, individually, to gauge a reaction. This approach can be useful at pinpointing your food allergies and sensitivities and is still considered the gold standard for determining which foods you may be sensitive to, even taking into account all of the advanced laboratory testing that is now available.

Elimination diets vary by approach, with some only avoiding the top eight most common food allergens—milk, eggs, fish, shellfish, tree nuts, peanuts, gluten, and soy—while other approaches are more comprehensive (such as the Autoimmune Protocol, discussed below). Some elimination diets call for avoiding a set of foods for a couple weeks before reintroduction; others go for trials that are a month or longer. The idea is that once your immune system has time off from a food, you are better able to gauge a reaction when you start eating it again.

We believe an elimination diet to be the ultimate tool to determine a set of foods that best support personal long-term healing. While, in theory, nutrient-dense diets such as Paleo are quite healthy to eat long-term, you may still find that you are sensitive to some of the included foods and getting to the root of those sensitivities can take healing to a whole new level.

THE AUTOIMMUNE PROTOCOL

The Autoimmune Protocol is an elimination and reintroduction protocol that has been specifically designed to help those with autoimmune disease determine their food allergies and sensitivities, reverse nutrient deficiencies, balance gut flora, and heal their bodies. The protocol has been developed and refined by Dr. Ballantyne and is outlined in detail in her book, *The Paleo*

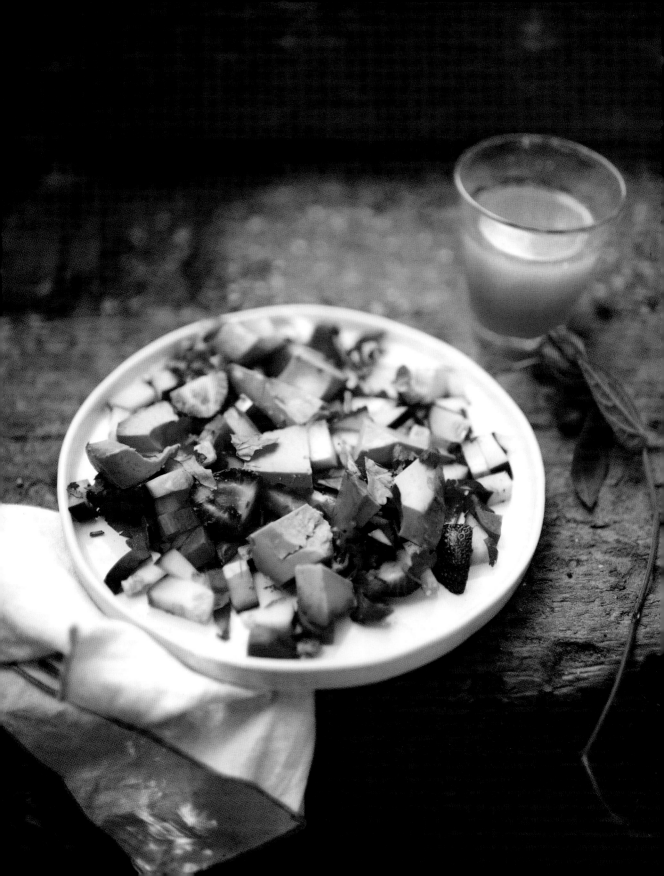

Approach. We believe this is the best and most specific elimination and reintroduction protocol for those with autoimmune disease, and following it gives you the opportunity to come up with your personalized healing diet.

In a nutshell, the Autoimmune Protocol calls for removing foods that are most likely to be problematic for people with autoimmune disease—grains, beans, legumes, dairy, eggs, nuts, seeds, and nightshades, as well as food chemicals and additives. In addition, nutrient-dense foods are added to restore nutrient status, such as bone broth, high-quality meat, and wild-caught fish, as well as organ meats, fermented foods, and a wide variety of fruits and vegetables. Over the course of the elimination phase (which can last from a month to a year), you take note of the changes you experience in your health. When it comes time to slowly and systematically reintroduce foods, you will be able to tell exactly which foods are holding you back and be prepared to use this information to construct a diet that will best support your healing needs.

The Autoimmune Protocol in Detail

In the last section, we gave you the Autoimmune Protocol in a nutshell, but in this section, we want to dive into the detail. The first thing to understand is that the Autoimmune Protocol is meant to serve as a template. Templates are preset formats that can easily be duplicated but, also *importantly*, can be adapted to individual uses. The Autoimmune Protocol is an elimination and reintroduction diet, but "diet" only in the sense that it refers to food intake. It is not a diet in the prescriptive, follow-the-rules sense. Diets of that nature are rigid and force people into molds that may not fit their needs. That one-size-fits-all approach to food is doomed to failure, since it leaves no room for the individual. On the other hand, a template promotes self-discovery through the use of an adaptable format. Depending on your genetics, your current level of health, your resources, and your goals, you can individualize this template to heal. By using the Autoimmune Protocol as your guide, you begin with a foundation that everyone can apply and from there, with careful self-experimentation, you discover the least-restricted diet that produces your best long-term health. The Autoimmune Protocol is not a set of commandments you desperately follow, hoping for a cookie-cutter result. It is a deliberate journey of healing wherein you blaze a unique trail.

A Two-Phased Process

The Autoimmune Protocol has two phases, an elimination phase and a reintroduction phase. During the elimination phase, remove the following from your diet (see the charts starting on page 64).

- Grains and pseudo-grains
- Beans and legumes
- Dairy
- Refined/processed seed and vegetable oils

- Eggs
- Alcohol
- Food chemicals
- Refined and alternative sweeteners
- Nuts and seeds
- Nightshade-family foods

Health can be boosted with the addition of the following nutrient-dense foods.

- Bone broth
- Grass-fed organ meats
- Grass-fed gelatin or collagen
- Oily, cold-water, wild-caught fish and shellfish
- Fermented foods or probiotic beverages
- A colorful array of fruits and vegetables

There are very specific reasons why these foods are intentionally excluded or included in the protocol, but we will not be going into that discussion here. For those who would like to do more research, we recommend reading *The Paleo Approach* by Dr. Ballantyne.

After good health is firmly reestablished, a four-part process of reintroducing foods can be attempted. (The details about reintroductions can be found on page 75). Everyone will need a minimum of 30 days in the elimination phase, many will need a few months, and some will need up to a year. The elimination phase is highly vari-

able because individual healing timelines are unique to each person. For example, the degree of severity of your autoimmune disease at the time you begin the protocol, how long your autoimmune disease went undiagnosed (as this may have contributed to the development of additional autoimmune diseases or organ damage), how nutrient deficient you are when you begin, and your personal commitment level to the process all affect the healing timeline.

Why Is the Autoimmune Protocol an Ideal Starting Point?

You may be wondering: Why is the Autoimmune Protocol such a good starting point for increased wellness when, in fact, there are so many other approaches out there?

1. IT REMOVES FOODS THAT MAY TRIGGER AN IMMUNE RESPONSE, ARE HARMFUL TO THE GUT, AND LEAD TO HORMONAL DYS-REGULATION. As you know from Chapter 1, autoimmune disease is all about an immune system that has gone awry. One of the common responses of our immune systems to perceived triggers is increased inflammation. With inflammation comes all sorts of aches, pains, and uncomfortable symptoms. These same potentially immune-provoking foods also damage our intestinal linings and lead to hormonal imbalance. By removing these foods, you essentially give your system a break. As it calms, inflammation subsides, damage heals, and hormones balance, and with those changes, all your discomfort diminishes. *The Autoimmune Protocol gives us a clean slate.*

2. IT RESTORES NUTRIENTS AND FLORA THAT PROMOTE A HEALTHY GUT AND WELL-REGULATED IMMUNE FUNCTION.

Micronutrient deficiencies are common in autoimmune disease. Many of us are deficient in fat-soluble vitamins (A, D, E, and K); minerals like zinc, iron, or magnesium; B vitamins, vitamin C, antioxidants, non-vitamin nutrients, and certain amino acids. In addition, a healthy balance of gut microorganisms is often severely disrupted. The foods we focus on in the Autoimmune Protocol are very nutrient dense, fueling healing and balancing our gut flora. Over time, this replenishment from foods rich in nutrients and probiotics greatly strengthens our systems. *The Autoimmune Protocol restores us.*

3. IT PROVIDES A FRAMEWORK FOR BUILDING A LIFELONG DIET EXACTLY SUITED TO YOU.

We've said it so many times already in this chapter, but it bears repeating: There is no one-size-fits-all diet. Fortunately, the Autoimmune Protocol provides a clean slate and restoration that allow us to move forward with an experimentation process that is clear. With all the "noise" of a damaged system silenced and proper functioning reestablished, you are able to take a structured approach to food that helps you discover what works best. *The Autoimmune Protocol empowers us.*

Taking the Plunge

The list of foods to avoid may be disheartening when you begin. The list of foods to include can also be very intimidating, because many of these foods are unfamiliar and don't often make a regular appearance in the modern diet. We want you to know that these feelings are quite normal. If after evaluating your current health and future wellness goals, you realize the Autoimmune Protocol is right for you, we encourage you to take the plunge. If you commit to this process of self-discovery, allowing for adequate healing time during the elimination phase, intentionally adding nutrient-packed foods, and committing to significant lifestyle improvements, the results usually make the process well worth the initial trepidation.

The Autoimmune Protocol also emphasizes high-quality food sources, abundant food variety, and a great deal of food preparation, but it is important to just get started with the transition (see page 72 for guidance). Over time, you can tweak your approach to maximize your time and financial resources to best undertake the process. Don't let perfection paralyze you. The Autoimmune Protocol provides a fantastic starting point for greatly increased wellness. If you put in the effort and work patiently to understand what your body needs, you will soon have a template that is personalized and promotes your best health.

Foods to Include

Meat

Beef	Goat	Rabbit
Bison	Lamb	Venison
Elk	Pork	

Poultry

Chicken	Goose	
Duck	Turkey	

Fish

Anchovy	Halibut	Snapper
Arctic char	Herring	Sole
Bass	Mackerel	Swordfish
Carp	Mahi-mahi	Tilapia
Catfish	Monkfish	Trout
Cod	Salmon	Tuna
Haddock	Sardine	

Shellfish

Clams	Mussels	Shrimp
Crab	Octopus	Snails
Crawfish	Oysters	Squid
Lobster	Scallops	

Animal fats

Bacon fat (if the ingredients are compliant)	Poultry fat (like duck or goose)	Strutto (clarified pork fat)
Lard (rendered pork back or kidney fat)	Schmaltz (rendered chicken or goose fat)	Tallow (rendered fat from beef or lamb)

Plant-based fats and oils

Avocado oil	Olive oil	Palm shortening
Coconut oil	Palm oil	Red palm oil

Vegetable-like fruits

Avocados	Olives	Summer squash (zucchini)
Cucumbers	Plantains	Winter squash (like butternut, delicata, and acorn)
Okra	Pumpkin	

The Autoimmune Wellness Handbook

Foods to Include (cont.)

Leafy green vegetables

Arugula	Collard greens	Mustard greens
Beet greens	Dandelion greens	Radicchio
Bok choy	Endive	Spinach
Brussels sprouts	Kale	Swiss chard
Cabbage	Lettuce	Turnip greens
Celery	Mizuna	Watercress

Root vegetables

Arrowroot	Horseradish	Tigernut
Beets	Jerusalem artichoke	Turmeric
Carrots	Jicama	Turnips
Cassava	Parsnips	Wasabi
Celeriac	Radishes	Water chestnuts
Daikon	Rutabagas	Yams
Garlic	Sweet potatoes	
Ginger	Taro	

Other vegetables

Artichokes	Chives	Rhubarb
Asparagus	Fennel	Seaweed (like arame, nori, wakame)
Broccoli	Leeks	
Cauliflower	Onions	Shallots

Fruit

Apples	Grapefruit	Peaches
Apricots	Grapes	Persimmons
Blackberries	Guava	Pineapple
Blueberries	Honeydew	Plantains
Cantaloupe	Huckleberries	Plums
Cherimoya	Kiwifruit	Pomegranate
Cherries	Lemons	Quince
Clementines	Limes	Raspberries
Coconut	Mangoes	Strawberries
Cranberries	Mulberries	Tamarind
Currants	Nectarines	Tangerines
Dates	Oranges	Watermelon
Durian	Papaya	
Figs	Passionfruit	

Foods to Include (cont.)

Probiotic foods

Fermented meat or fish	Kvass	Nondairy kefir (made with fruit)
Kombucha	Lacto-fermented fruits and vegetables	Sauerkraut

Edible fungi/mushrooms

Chanterelle	Oyster	Shiitake
Cremini	Porcini	Truffle
Morel	Portobello	

Herbs and spices

Asafetida	Garlic	Rosemary
Basil	Ginger	Saffron
Bay leaf	Horseradish	Sage
Chamomile	Kaffir lime leaf	Savory leaf
Chervil	Lavender	Spearmint
Chive	Lemon balm	Tarragon
Cilantro (coriander leaf)	Lemongrass	Tea (both green and black; check herbal teas for nightshades and seeds)
Cinnamon	Mace	
Clove	Marjoram	Thyme
Curry leaf	Oregano	Turmeric
Dillweed	Parsley	Vanilla (whole)
Fennel leaf	Peppermint	

Other cooking ingredients

Apple cider vinegar	Coconut concentrate (otherwise known as butter, manna, or cream)	Fish sauce
Balsamic vinegar		Olives
Capers		Red wine vinegar
Carob powder	Coconut milk	Sea salt
Coconut aminos	Coconut vinegar	White wine vinegar

Occasional sweeteners

Coconut sugar	Honey	Maple syrup
Coconut syrup	Maple sugar	Molasses

The Autoimmune Wellness Handbook

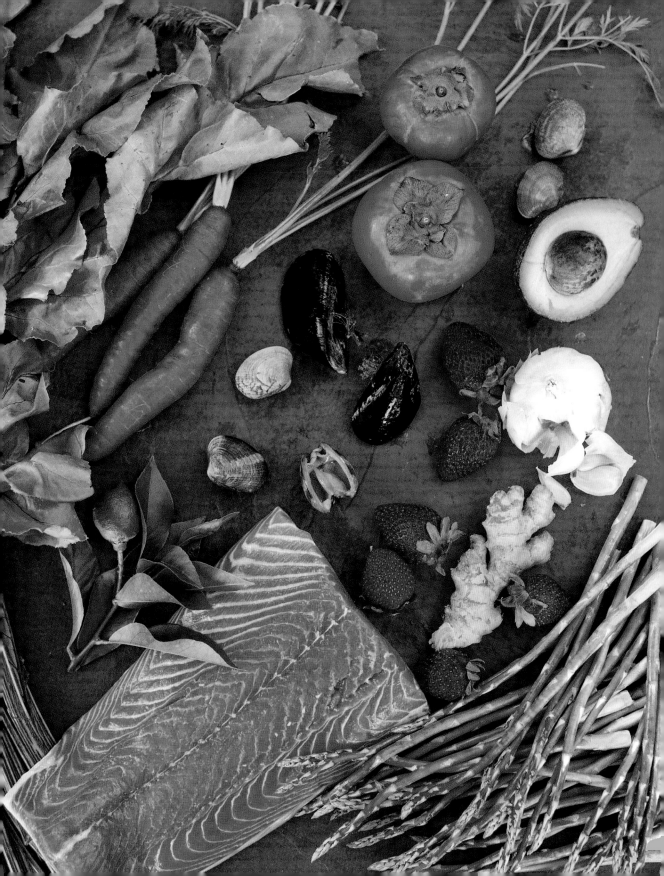

Foods to Avoid

Grains and pseudo-grains

Amaranth	Millet	Sorghum
Barley	Oats	Spelt
Buckwheat	Quinoa	Teff
Corn	Rice	Triticale
Kamut	Rye	Wheat

Beans and legumes

Adzuki beans	Green beans	Peanuts
Black beans	Kidney beans	Peas
Black-eyed peas	Lentils	Pinto beans
Cannellini beans	Lima beans	Soybeans (including soy products like tofu)
Chickpeas	Mung beans	
Fava beans	Navy beans	

Dairy (bovine, goat, or from other species)

Butter	Ghee	Sour cream
Buttermilk	Ice cream	Whey
Cottage cheese	Kefir	Whipping cream
Cream	Milk	Yogurt

Industrial seed and vegetable oils

Canola oil	Palm kernel oil	Soybean oil
Corn oil	Peanut oil	Sunflower oil
Cottonseed oil	Safflower oil	

Eggs

Chicken eggs	Duck eggs	Other species

Sugar alcohols and non-nutritive sweeteners

Acesulfame potassium	Neotame	Sucralose
Aspartame	Saccharin	Xylitol
Erythritol	Sorbitol	
Mannitol	Stevia	

Foods to Avoid (cont.)

Alcohol

All alcohol

Food chemicals

Artificial and natural flavors	Monosodium glutamate (MSG)	Textured vegetable protein
Artificial coloring	Nitrites or nitrates (naturally occurring are okay)	Trans fats
Carrageenan		Xanthan gum
Guar gum	Phosphoric acid	Yeast extract
Lecithin	Propylene glycol	Any ingredient names you don't recognize

Nuts (including flours, butters, or oils derived from them)

Almonds	Hazelnuts	Pistachios
Brazil nuts	Macadamia nuts	Walnuts
Cashews	Pecans	
Chestnuts	Pine nuts	

Seeds (including flours, butters, spices, or oils derived from them)

Anise	Cumin	Nutmeg
Caraway	Dill seed	Poppy
Celery seed	Fennel seed	Pumpkin
Chia	Fenugreek	Sesame
Cocoa	Flax	Sunflower
Coffee	Hemp	
Coriander	Mustard seed	

Nightshade-family foods (including products and spices derived from them)

Ashwagandha	Goji berries	Tomatillos
Bell peppers	Hot peppers	Tomatoes
Cayenne pepper	Paprika	
Eggplant	Potatoes	

Fruit and berry spices

Allspice	Cardamom	Pepper (black, green, pink, or white)
Anise	Juniper	
Caraway		

NUTRIENT DENSITY

The biggest mistake you can make in adopting the Autoimmune Protocol is overlooking the concept of nutrient density. It's easy to get lost in eliminations, but of equal importance is replacing the removed foods with those that have the nutrients needed to reverse deficiencies and heal the body.

Common nutrient deficiencies in the modern diet include the B vitamins (especially B_{12}); the fat-soluble vitamins A, D, E, and K; minerals like magnesium, calcium, and iron; antioxidants like vitamin C; essential fatty acids EPA and DHA; fiber that feeds our gut flora; and the amino acids that make up our structure and perform functions throughout our bodies. Luckily, the Autoimmune Protocol focuses on including nutritional powerhouse foods, like organ meats (especially liver—check out our recipes on pages 173 and 189), bone broth (page 168), fermented vegetables (page 174), oily, cold-water fish and shellfish, and a wide variety of colorful fruits and vegetables. You might be surprised to find your healing accelerated and your energy dramatically increased after eating these powerful foods.

On the next page, we have provided a chart to help you to compare the nutrient density of some key foods so you can choose which ones to prioritize in your diet. You will find the most nutrient-packed foods at the top of the list. Making sure to include them as often as you are able gives you the best opportunity to heal.

It may be tempting to seek out supplements instead of focusing on eating these nutritional powerhouse foods, but our experience is that getting nutrition from food is always ideal. Nature has packaged these nutrients in the easiest way for your body to assimilate them—containing the necessary cofactors and macronutrients required for proper digestion and absorption. If you are working with a practitioner, you may find that some smart supplementation speeds the process early on, but be sure to review your diet as well.

MICKEY'S EXPERIENCE

I believe incorporating nutrient density when I embarked on the Autoimmune Protocol was one of the early keys to my success in healing my body. Prior to this way of eating, I had followed a vegan diet (no animal products) for more than a decade and was suffering from severe nutritional deficiencies that were not responding to supplementation. When I embarked on the elimination diet, I was sure to include lots of nutrient-dense foods like bone broth, beef liver, salmon, and fermented vegetables, and I believe these foods helped me to make quick progress. In fact, including beef liver pâté (see my recipe on page 173!) weekly for a month helped to reverse my anemia so quickly that my doctor believed my prior bloodwork to be in error!

Nutrient Powerhouses

Organ meats

Vitamin A	Vitamin B_{12}	Choline
Vitamin B_1	Vitamin D	Iron
Vitamin B_2	Vitamin K	Selenium
Vitamin B_3	Folate	Zinc
Vitamin B_6	Pantothenic acid	Copper

Broth

Calcium	Phosphorus	Collagen
Magnesium	Gelatin	

Oily fish

Vitamin D	EPA and DHA	Selenium
Vitamin B_{12}	Phosphorus	

Shellfish

Iron	Copper	Phosphorus
Zinc	Selenium	Iodine

Fermented foods

Probiotics	Vitamin K	

Leafy green vegetables

Vitamin K	Magnesium	Calcium
Folate	Insoluble fiber	Vitamin E
Manganese	Antioxidants	

Colorful fruits and vegetables

Vitamin C	Antioxidants	Fiber

DIETARY TRANSITION

Transition Styles

Making a big change in any area of our lives is difficult. Everyone knows it is hard to learn new ways of doing things and even harder to drop old habits. Deciding on the best method for transitioning can be just as tough, especially when it comes to a shift in something as fundamental as the way we eat. There are plenty of expert opinions about the best way to handle dietary transition, but there isn't a ton of solid research that tells us for sure what the absolute best way is for long-term success. It comes down to knowing yourself well. Understanding your personality and realistically evaluating your lifestyle are the most important factors in choosing a transition method.

Once you've decided to change your diet, you have two options.

1. COLD TURKEY—If you know you thrive with a rip-off-the-Band-Aid approach, cold turkey might be best for you. Maybe you are great at envisioning your goals and steadfastly taking on a challenge. Cold turkey requires a great deal of self-motivation.

2. SLOW AND STEADY—Many people immediately rebel at the thought of such a drastic change to their familiar patterns. Maybe an all-or-nothing approach feels scary or makes you certain you'll fail. Baby steps can be an effective method for dietary transition. Slow and steady requires a high level of endurance.

Do you feel like there are times when you are both cold turkey and slow and steady? Most of us feel that way. Next, you'll find a self-test designed to help you pinpoint your transition style. Once you know the best method, you can start implementing some healing dietary changes.

Cold-Turkey Transition Guide

If you've determined that a fast transition is best suited to you, we recommend a 3-day jump-start process. You'll start with a weekend of planning and preparation. The focus will be to do as much as possible to get prepared for a Monday morning transition to the full-elimination phase of the Autoimmune Protocol.

- **FRIDAY**—Plan a menu and shopping list for the week ahead with all the foods to avoid eliminated and nutrient-dense foods included, using the meal plan starting on page 225, if needed. Clear out your pantry using the exercise on page 236.

- **SATURDAY**—Shop for foods necessary for your menu (you may find the shopping list starting on page 232 helpful here). Be sure to focus on bringing in as many Autoimmune Protocol–compliant ingredients as possible, so that you feel fully capable of maintaining the diet once you begin.

- **SUNDAY**—Batch-cook to prepare for the week ahead. This means cooking multiple dishes to eat as leftovers or use as components of quick meals throughout the week. Great batch-cooking recipes include broths, soups, stews, roasted meats, and

WHICH WAY WILL WORK FOR YOU?

Here are a few questions to ask yourself when considering which transition approach is best for you.

COLD TURKEY

☐ Am I willing to make substantial changes to my schedule in order to prioritize healing?

☐ Am I child-free or do I have older children who won't be strongly impacted by this process?

☐ Do I feel ready to commit immediately?

☐ Do I have strong planning and preparation skills?

☐ Do I know my way around the kitchen?

☐ Am I at a point with my disease where I need relief as quickly as possible?

☐ Do I have a partner or a family member who will support me through a rapid transition?

☐ Do I have a history of successfully diving into big changes?

☐ Am I willing and able to prioritize my budget to focus on food immediately?

SLOW AND STEADY

☐ Do I have an extremely busy schedule with little flexibility?

☐ Do I have young children or other family members who may not be adopting this diet?

☐ Is full commitment something I normally need to take time to consider?

☐ Do I prefer to take on planning and preparation tasks in phases?

☐ Will I need time to learn my way around the kitchen?

☐ Does the stress of a rapid transition seem more uncomfortable than my disease symptoms?

☐ Will the process be difficult for my partner and require more time for him/her as I make adjustments?

☐ Do I find myself repeatedly trying to make all-or-nothing changes and failing?

☐ Do I have a very tight budget without much room to reallocate funds to groceries quickly?

some vegetable sides. You might also consider using Sunday to reach out to a few key family members or friends and ask for support for your upcoming transition.

Slow-and-Steady Transition Guide

If you've determined that a slow-and-steady transition is best suited to you, we recommend a 6-week process. You'll start with a weeklong planning and preparation phase, which includes seeking support, and then use the next 5 weeks to tackle 2 food group eliminations per week, while also adding 1 new nutritional powerhouse. The eliminations with the greatest impact on your health are up first, and the eliminations with the least impact are last; this gives you some bang for your buck early in the process and hopefully adds to your motivation. The end result will be compliance with the full-elimination phase of the Autoimmune Protocol.

Week 1

- Ask a few family members or friends to offer you encouragement as you transition your diet.

- Plan a menu and shopping list for next week eliminating all **GRAINS** and **ALCOHOL** and including **HEALTHY FATS**, like olive oil, coconut oil, and solid cooking fat (see recipe on page 170).

- Shop for the foods necessary according to your menu.

- At the end of the week, remove all **GRAINS** and **ALCOHOL** from your house in preparation for next week.

- Do one batch-cooking session to prepare your meals for next week.

Week 2

- This week, start avoiding **GRAINS** and **ALCOHOL** in your diet, and start adding **HEALTHY FATS**, following the menu you prepared last week.

- Plan a menu and shopping list for next week eliminating all **LEGUMES** and **NIGHTSHADES** and including **BONE BROTH** (see recipe on page 168).

- Shop for the foods necessary according to your menu.

- At the end of the week, remove all **LEGUMES** and **NIGHTSHADES** from your house in preparation for next week.

- Do one batch-cooking session to prepare your meals for next week.

Week 3

- This week, start avoiding **LEGUMES** and **NIGHTSHADES** in your diet, and start adding **BONE BROTH**, following the menu you prepared last week.

- Plan a menu and shopping list for next week eliminating all **DAIRY** and **COFFEE** and including **PROBIOTIC DRINKS** (see Resources on page 261).

- Shop for the foods necessary according to your menu.

- At the end of the week, remove all **DAIRY** and **COFFEE** from your house in preparation for next week.

- Do one batch-cooking session to prepare your meals for next week.

Week 4

- This week, start avoiding **DAIRY** and **COFFEE** in your diet, and start adding **PROBIOTIC DRINKS**, following the menu you prepared last week.

- Plan a menu and shopping list for next week eliminating all **FOOD ADDITIVES**, **REFINED/PROCESSED SUGARS**, **EGGS**, and **REFINED/PROCESSED OILS** and including **FERMENTED FOODS** (see recipe on page 174).

- Shop for the foods necessary according to your menu.

- At the end of the week, remove all **FOOD ADDITIVES**, **REFINED/PROCESSED SUGARS**, **EGGS**, and **REFINED/PROCESSED OILS** from your house in preparation for next week.

- Do one batch-cooking session to prepare your meals for next week.

Week 5

- This week, start avoiding **EGGS**, **REFINED/PROCESSED SUGARS**, **REFINED/PROCESSED OILS**, and **FOOD ADDITIVES** in your diet, and start adding **FERMENTED FOODS**, following the menu you prepared last week.

- Plan a menu and shopping list for next week eliminating all **NUTS**, **SEEDS**, and **FRUIT- AND BERRY-BASED SPICES** and including **ORGAN MEATS** (see recipe on page 173).

- Shop for the foods necessary according to your menu.

- At the end of the week, remove all **NUTS**, **SEEDS**, and **FRUIT- AND BERRY-BASED SPICES** from your house in preparation for next week.

- Do one batch-cooking session to prepare your meals for next week.

Week 6

- This week, start avoiding **NUTS**, **SEEDS**, and **FRUIT- AND BERRY-BASED SPICES** in your diet, and start adding **ORGAN MEATS** following the menu you prepared last week.

- As of this week, you are compliant with the full-elimination phase of the Autoimmune Protocol!

- Continue to use meal planning and batch-cooking as you maintain your elimination phase.

REINTRODUCTIONS

Reintroducing Foods

The elimination phase of the Autoimmune Protocol is not meant to be followed long-term—the next, and equally important, phase is called *reintroduction*. Through a slow and systematic process of putting foods on trial that you avoided on the elimination diet, you will find out if any food allergies or sensitivities are potentially contributing to your symptoms. This is a delicate but informative process that requires you to learn how to access your own inner wisdom about the cause and effect of what you put into your body. The end product is the least-restricted diet that is most supportive of your long-term healing, one that gives you the best chance of success without driving you crazy.

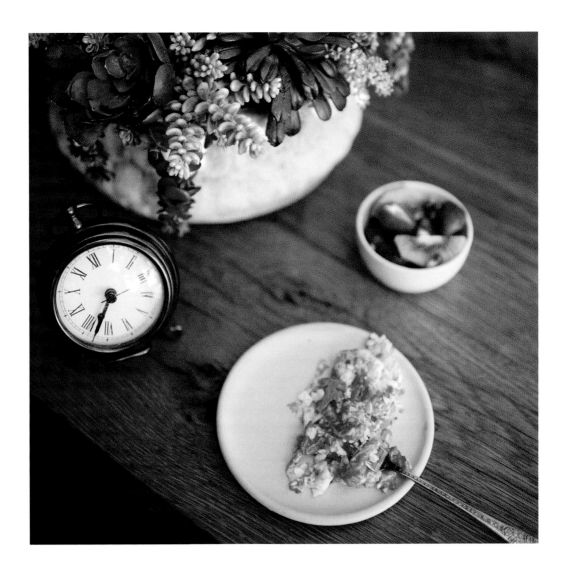

How Long Do You Stay on the Elimination Diet?

Before you decide to reintroduce foods, you need to assess whether you have done the elimination phase long enough, with 100 percent compliance. Initially, you may want to give yourself a goal of 30 days, and then make a reassessment if you'd like to

continue on longer at that point—it is hard to gauge at the beginning of the process how it will go for your unique situation. Sometimes, people feel initial improvements (such as better digestion, energy, and clearer skin) in 30 days but wish to proceed for 60 to 90 days to see if they continue to progress upward. Others may see a dramatic reversal of symptoms in that 30-day period, making them great candidates for reintroduction sooner rather than later. Your experience on the elimination diet is going to depend on a lot of factors—your state of health going in, autoimmune conditions, degree of tissue damage, and starting nutritional status. How long to stay on the elimination diet varies from person to person, and advice from your key player might also be useful here.

When Are You Ready to Reintroduce Foods?

You are ready to reintroduce foods when you have seen *measurable* improvements during the elimination phase. This can be general health improvements, like better sleep, less pain, or mental clarity, or specific improvements, like a lessening of your autoimmune symptoms. Which improvements you see aren't as important as the fact that they are there, and that they are clear—if you don't have an improved baseline to compare with when you start to reintroduce foods, you won't learn much. If you are not experiencing any changes after 30 to 90 days on the Autoimmune Protocol, you will want to check out our troubleshooting section on page 85 or enlist the help of your key player to look for underlying root causes that are acting as roadblocks to your success.

Why Is It Important to Reintroduce Foods?

It is common to see a lot of improvements and sometimes a full reversal of symptoms while on the elimination diet. When this is the case for you, it may be tempting to think "well, maybe I will continue to eat this way forever!" While some people find that they are not able to successfully reintroduce many foods, it is more common to be able to tolerate some of the foods in the first stages of reintroduction (which we will cover in the following section). Especially when you are experiencing success, reintroduction is an *essential* part of the Autoimmune Protocol. Successful reintroductions expand the list of foods you can eat, making your diet less restrictive and easier to integrate into your life over the long-term. While it is not advised to reintroduce foods when you haven't experienced success (see the troubleshooting guide on page 85), you can and *should* start reintroducing foods when you start to feel better!

Reintroduction Protocol

We know it's tempting to start eating all of the foods you have eliminated right away after experiencing success, but embarking on the reintroduction process carefully ensures that you don't have to start over! This is a very delicate process and not to be rushed. The more systematic you are about reintroductions, the easier it is going to be to make an assessment about whether or not a food is in or out. Familiarize yourself with the reintroduction protocol as well as the stages of reintroduction *before* you get there, so that you know what to expect.

The protocol for reintroductions, as outlined by Dr. Sarah Ballantyne in *The Paleo Approach,* is the following:

1. Pick a food to challenge and get ready to eat it a couple of times in 1 day.

2. Eat the food for the first time, only having a nibble. Wait 15 minutes, and if you don't have any symptoms, take a small bite, a little larger than the last.

3. Wait another 15 minutes, and if you still don't have any symptoms, take another bite, again slightly larger.

4. Wait 2 to 3 hours, watching to see if symptoms appear.

5. Next, eat an average quantity of the food, either by itself or as part of a meal.

6. Watch your symptoms for 3 to 7 days afterward, being sure to avoid the food you reintroduced as well as not reintroducing any other foods.

7. You may incorporate that food into your diet if you have no symptoms during this whole process.

This protocol may seem overly cautious, but it is the safest way to reintroduce foods after a long period of elimination. During the time you have avoided potential triggers, your body becomes less inflamed and your immune system gets a break from the constant attack. Sometimes, even when you reintroduce a food you used to eat all the time, you may be surprised to feel an obvious reaction. Many of us have been here before! To avoid unnecessary setbacks, it is important to take this reintroduction process slowly and methodically, even if you suspect that a food is not a problem going into the process.

Journaling is an invaluable tool when going through the reintroductions. It helps you recognize symptoms and patterns that might indicate the source of a food reaction that would be otherwise hard to gauge. We have included a sample journal page on page 81 to help you get started.

In What Order Do You Reintroduce Foods?

When deciding which foods to reintroduce and when, it may be tempting to try the

ANGIE'S EXPERIENCE

Reintroductions can be such a confusing process! When I first began attempting them, I wasn't really sure what signs or symptoms I should be looking for that might indicate I was sensitive to a food, or more happily, that I could begin including it in my diet again. Dr. Sarah Ballantyne's guidance on the topic wasn't yet published, but to my surprise, as I undertook the process, I was able to discern my body's communication. It was like all the "noise" I'd previously been hearing was silenced and signs of sensitivity were so much easier to spot. One example was when I first attempted to reintroduce white potatoes, a nightshade vegetable. The next morning, I woke with searing pain in my hip joints. This had been something I lived with all the time prior to the elimination diet and it made it clear to me that I was still sensitive. The good news is that with several more months of healing, I no longer got the joint pain. I can eat homemade French fries without fear these days!

Reintroduction Stages

STAGE I	egg yolks, legumes with edible pods, fruit- and berry-based spices, seed-based spices, seed and nut oils, ghee from grass-fed dairy
STAGE II	seeds, nuts (except cashews and pistachios), cocoa or chocolate, egg whites, grass-fed butter, alcohol (in small quantities)
STAGE III	cashews and pistachios, eggplant, sweet peppers, paprika, coffee, grass-fed raw cream, fermented grass-fed raw dairy (yogurt and kefir)
STAGE IV	other dairy products (grass-fed whole milk and cheese), chile peppers, tomatoes, potatoes, other nightshades and nightshade spices, alcohol (in larger quantities), white rice, traditionally prepared legumes (soaked and fermented), traditionally prepared gluten-free grains (soaked and fermented)

foods you are craving the most first—perhaps grains, tomatoes, wine, or cheese. However, it is important to choose the order of reintroduction carefully to avoid a flare or setback. Not all foods avoided during the elimination phase of the Autoimmune Protocol carry an equal potential to be problematic, so it is best to start with foods that are *least* likely to cause a problem before working into the category of *most* likely to cause a problem.

Dr. Ballantyne has categorized the foods in reintroduction stages, starting with those that are least likely to cause a problem. We recommend starting with the foods in stage I and only moving on to the next stage after you have a few successful reintroductions under your belt. While you may find some foods you are sensitive to in the early stages, they are less likely to produce strong reactions that can cause a major setback. The foods in the later stages, III and IV, are most difficult to reintroduce.

What Kinds of Reactions Are You Looking For?

When reintroducing foods, you want to be aware of all of the potential reactions you could have and ready to take note of them in your journal (see page 81). Reactions can range from severe and obvious to subtle and unclear. After going through the process of elimination, it is possible to react to foods you may have been eating on a regular basis before you started your elimination. Because of this, you need to be aware of the potential reactions you could have—some of them may surprise you!

- **RETURN OR WORSENING OF AUTOIMMUNE SYMPTOMS**—If you experienced relief from your autoimmune symptoms while in the elimination phase, look for signs that they could be coming back (for instance, joint pain for rheumatoid arthritis, or a rash for psoriasis).

- **DIGESTIVE CHANGES**—Subtle or obvious changes, depending on how your digestion functioned before the elimination phase, can be a bad sign. You want to be on the lookout for things like heartburn, constipation, diarrhea, stomach pain, gas, bloating, or burping when reintroducing foods.

- **HEADACHES, RACING PULSE, OR DIZZINESS**—These can be common warning signs of food sensitivities.

- **FATIGUE**—Check in with your energy levels when going through the reintroduction process. Although this can be a tricky one to pinpoint, some people feel a return of exhaustion when reintroducing certain foods.

- **SLEEP DISTURBANCES**—Trouble falling asleep, staying asleep, or waking up throughout the night can be a sign that a food is problematic.

- **JOINT OR MUSCLE PAIN**—Increased joint or muscle pain, especially with certain foods like those in the nightshade family, can be common with food sensitivities.

- **SKIN CHANGES**—Anything from flushing to rashes, hives, itchiness, or acne indicates an issue. Pay attention to your skin and if there are any changes to it as you reintroduce foods.

- **MOOD CHANGES**—Although many are surprised when they encounter this reaction, some can feel anxiety, depression, or other mood changes (like anger, tearfulness, or rage) when they are sensitive to a food.

What If You Can't Tell If You Are Reacting to a Food?

If you have done the elimination diet with 100 percent compliance, seen measurable improvement, and are having a hard time telling if your food reintroductions are successful or not, it is sometimes helpful to take a slower approach to reintroduction. Instead of taking 3 to 7 days between reintroductions, give yourself 1 to 2 weeks to see if anything crops up over the long term. Having added fewer variables into the mix, it will be easier to note reactions.

What If You Have a Really Bad Reaction to a Food?

Hopefully, if you reintroduce foods in the order we advise (see the stages on page 79) and start with the foods you are *least* likely to react to, you won't have a severe response. However, this can happen, and if you find yourself in this situation, you need to go back to the full-elimination phase to recover. Once you have returned to the level of health you were at when you started reintroducing foods, you can try again with a different food. If you encounter a reaction that is particularly severe, this may be a good indicator that this food will not work for your body long-term.

The Autoimmune Wellness Handbook

If You React to a Food, Does That Mean You Can Never Eat It Again?

You may find that you react to many foods early on in the process, but as your gut health, nutrient status, and general well-being improve, you may tolerate more foods over time. This is why it is important to continue to reintroduce foods over the long-term and not operate on the assumption that nothing will change. Reacting to a lot of early-stage foods may mean that you need some more time in the elimination phase, letting your body do some healing before trying them again.

That being said, there may be some reintroductions that may not be possible for you, at least if you want to continue to see the benefits of being on the Autoimmune Protocol. Later-stage foods like dairy, nightshades, and grains can be a lifelong problem for some, but it is up to the individual to see where he or she lies on the spectrum of tolerance and if those foods are supporting healing.

Reintroduction Journal Sample Pages

It is important to keep a journal when reintroducing foods so that you don't have to rely on memory alone to evaluate your trials and successes. The more information you are able to track here, the better. This sample journal page can be used for the trial of a specific food or to track your daily consumption and note any symptoms.

Journal Page

Date: _____

Sample Day

Time: _____

Food: _____

Time: _____

Food: _____

Time: _____

Food: _____

Time: _____

Food: _____

Today's notes:

Physical changes: _____

_____

_____

_____

_____

Emotional changes: _____

_____

_____

_____

_____

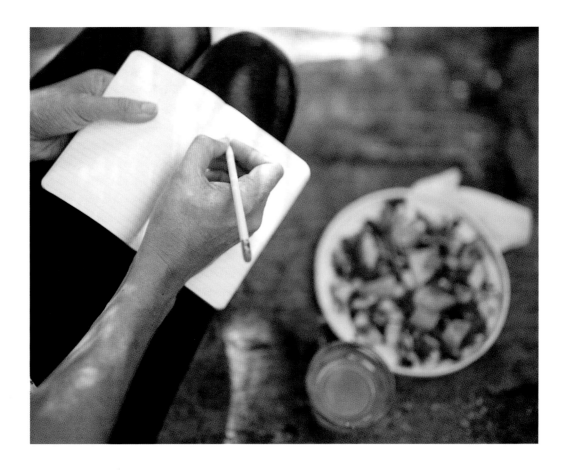

BALANCE

Finding Balance

It is no surprise that many of us have had long, difficult, potentially even traumatic experiences with our autoimmune diseases. We may have tried numerous approaches to healing or symptom management, from medications to fad diets. The journey can be fraught with mental and emotional struggles and balance, especially in terms of diet, often seems unattainable.

When we speak about balance here, we mean finding the sweet spot where you are no more food restricted than is absolutely necessary for your personal best health and you are enjoying a healthy relationship with food. You may find yourself vulnerable to losing perspective and spiraling into uncompromising, even harmful, food relationships when adopting food-elimination protocols. In the beginning, this process may go unnoticed. In your attempt to heal, you may find that certain food eliminations help alleviate symptoms and perhaps even have added benefits like a more slender physique or clearer skin. Your thoughts move in the direction of "more is better," and before the pattern is even recognized, unnecessary levels of restriction may have led to intense anxiety around food and disordered eating.

We absolutely believe in the healing power of food. We know the Autoimmune Protocol can have an enormous impact on the foundations of good health and is not "disordered eating," but the line between food as medicine versus food as fear can be difficult to discern for some. Our hope is that with mindfulness and self-awareness, we can all approach healing with diet and lifestyle with a spirit of enjoyment and transformation. This journey is about restoring our best selves, not developing burdened hearts and minds. In the following pages, you'll find more detailed explorations on maintaining balance.

Food Fears and Disordered Eating

You might confront food-related fears on your path with the Autoimmune Protocol. Food fear can be a temporary issue you learn to quickly overcome or a severe clinical disorder that significantly impacts or even threatens your life. Fears might have a legitimate basis in a life-threatening allergy on one end of the spectrum but range to harmful impaired thinking on the other. If you think your patterns are verging on severe and not as easily addressed as less-complex fears, there are ways to get help.

Clinically recognized eating disorders have a variety of signs and symptoms. There are also eating disturbances that are not classified, but have much in common with the recognized disorders. If you notice yourself edging toward an unhealthy place or if you have struggled with disordered eating in the past and recognize yourself being triggered into old, harmful patterns, please seek help. There are many trained professionals who can assist you in addressing these serious issues. You can start by contacting the National Eating Disorders Association, The Alliance for Eating Disorders Awareness, or using Eating Disorder Hope's directory to find many other organizations that are ready to help.

How Long Do You Need to Eat This Way?

We've said it several times already in this chapter, but a few more repetitions won't hurt—you are not meant to eat according to the elimination phase of the Autoimmune Protocol long-term. A strict elimination *phase* allows your system to calm and a "wellness baseline" to be established. Depending on many factors, your elimination phase may be longer or shorter than others' before you attempt *reintroductions*. The key words here are *phase* and *reintroductions*. The goal is the least-restricted diet that supports wellness and allows you to live a full life (without crazy-making food rules to follow forever!).

Now for some generalizations, because having some basic guidance helps.

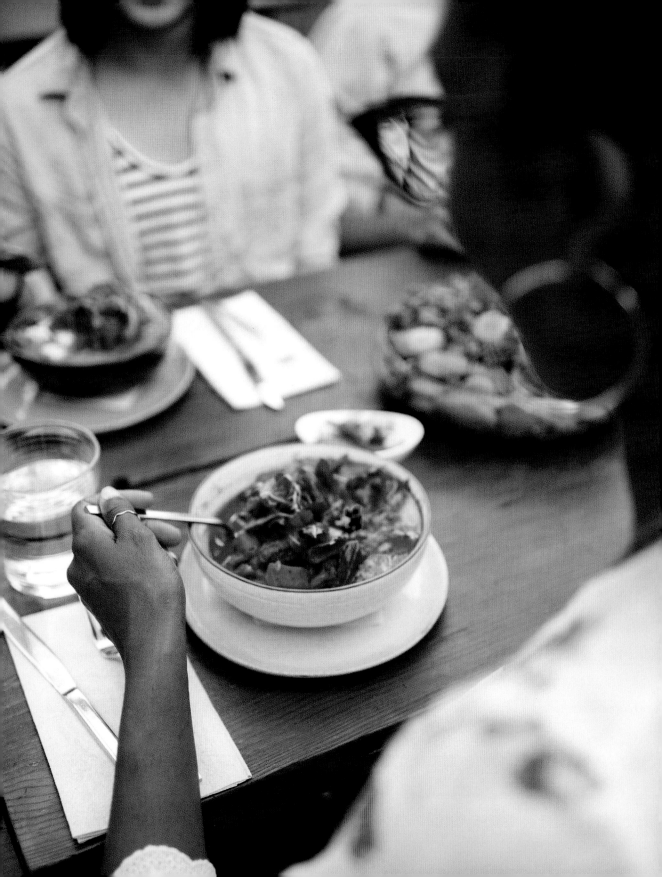

- Everyone does a minimum of 30 days in the elimination phase.

- Many reach best results with a bit longer time frame, usually 60 to 90 days.

- For some, improvements are not quite enough after 90 days. For this set, some troubleshooting and help from their key player can uncover underlying issues that require treatment beyond dietary and lifestyle changes (see next column). Remaining in elimination phase while working on these root issues can be helpful, since it removes variables.

- The vast majority do not need to remain in elimination phase beyond a year, even if they are continuing to explore root issues.

The important takeaway here is that once you've experienced successful healing, you can and *should* start expanding your diet. We all agree that chocolate is worth it!

Achieving Wellness, Not an Image

Your health is a precious gift. That is such a cliché statement, but those of us who have experienced the depths of autoimmune disease have had this dramatically demonstrated in our own lives. Enjoying robust health in a fully functioning body is unfortunately something very easily taken for granted, until you no longer have it. Having perfect hair, flawless skin, and a model's shape pales in comparison to an intestine that can absorb nutrients, a heart that can maintain rhythm, or lungs that can expand with life-giving oxygen.

Everyone wants to be seen as attractive, but if you make achieving wellness the primary motivator of this process, not a certain number on the scale or reflection in the mirror, you will benefit greatly from the balance that comes with that focus. In time, the work you have done to restore health and the deep appreciation you have for it will shine in unexpected ways. That kind of vitality is something everyone notices!

TROUBLESHOOTING

Sometimes, despite your best efforts, there may be something holding you back from experiencing the benefits of the elimination phase. In this section, we have outlined some areas you may want to explore should you find yourself not improving 30 to 90 days post transition. Support from your key player can be useful here, as testing, treatment, and expert guidance can help you navigate these complex situations.

Small Intestine Bacterial Overgrowth

When the beneficial bacteria that should reside in the large intestine (colon) migrate up into parts of the small intestine, a condition called **SMALL INTESTINE BACTERIAL OVERGROWTH** (SIBO) occurs. These bacteria wreak havoc on the digestive process by consuming food that should be absorbed into your body and produce hydrogen and methane gas as an end product. You end up with burping, gas, bloating, diarrhea, and constipation.

The bacteria that are involved in SIBO consume foods rich in short-chain fermentable carbohydrates, oligosaccharides, disaccharides, monosaccharides, and polyols (otherwise known as FODMAPs). Many commonly eaten foods contain these FODMAPs—onions, garlic, apples, and avocados to name a few. While healthy individuals are likely to feel no difference eating some of these foods, those suffering from SIBO may feel an exacerbation of their symptoms like bloating, abdominal pain, or stool changes.

SIBO is a common condition for those suffering from complex health issues like autoimmune disease, and successful treatment can provide benefit in many areas. While avoiding FODMAPs can be helpful in managing some of the symptoms caused by SIBO, you will need treatment (prescription or herbal antimicrobials) to eradicate it for good. We don't recommend attempting to self-manage or treat suspected SIBO without a practitioner. That being said, trying an elimination of FODMAPs for a couple of weeks can help you assess if your continuing digestive symptoms may be caused by this issue. If so, you can take this information to your key player and request to be tested for SIBO.

For more information about testing, treatment, and recovery from SIBO, we recommend the book *Digestive Health with Real Food* by Aglaée Jacob.

Low-FODMAP/Autoimmune Protocol

The list on page 87 includes high- and moderate-risk foods that also overlap with foods included during the elimination phase of the Autoimmune Protocol. If you have been diagnosed with or suspect SIBO, you may want to experiment with eliminating these foods and reintroducing according to a schedule defined by your practitioner's suggestions, as it can vary with treatment. You will find the foods on this list to be in two categories, denoting how potentially problematic they are for someone with SIBO. The word in parentheses next to the food is the fermentable sugar contained within.

A couple important notes: Not everyone with SIBO reacts to all foods in every category, so while you may tolerate avocados, another person with SIBO may not. Another thing to keep in mind is quantity: Sometimes you can get away with eating a small quantity of a certain food before experiencing symptoms. This is another place where diligent journaling can be a helpful practice.

Histamine Intolerance

HISTAMINE is a chemical produced by the body or contained in food that is a neurotransmitter (hormonal messenger), as well as a part of the body's inflammatory response. Under normal conditions, it is broken down and detoxified in the gut. Some people have HISTAMINE INTOLERANCE, a condition where their bodies cannot handle the excess histamine. This can cause symptoms such as headaches and migraines, flushing, rashes, hives, congestion, racing

High-FODMAP Foods List

AVOID

Vegetables

Artichokes (fructose)	Jerusalem artichokes (fructan)	Raddichio (fructan)
Asparagus (fructose)	Leeks (fructan)	Shallots (fructan)
Cabbage (fructan)	Okra (fructan)	
Garlic (fructan)	Onions (fructan)	

Fruit

Apples (fructose and polyol)	Fruit juice (fructose)	Pears (polyol)
Apricots (polyol)	Grapes (fructose)	Persimmons (polyol)
Blackberries (polyol)	Mangos (fructose)	Plums (polyol)
Cherries (fructose and polyol)	Nectarines (polyol)	Watermelon (polyol)
Dried fruit (fructose)	Peaches (polyol)	

Sweeteners

Honey

BE CAUTIOUS

Vegetables

Avocados (polyol)	Butternut squash (fructan)	Mushrooms (polyol)
Beets (fructan)	Cauliflower (polyol)	Sauerkraut (fructan)
Broccoli (fructan)	Celery (polyol)	Sweet potatoes (polyol)
Brussels sprouts (fructan)	Fennel bulb (fructan)	Yams (polyol)

Fruit

Bananas, unripe	Lychee (polyol)
Longan (polyol)	Rambutan (polyol)

Sweeteners

Coconut flour	Dried coconut
Coconut milk	Maple syrup
Coconut sugar	

High-Histamine Foods List

Foods on the Autoimmune Protocol and common reintroductions that are also high in histamine include:

- Alcohol (even when cooked off)
- Canned fish
- Canned meat
- Cheese
- Coconut aminos
- Cured meat (bacon, sausage, lunchmeat)
- Dried fruit
- Fermented vegetables (including sauerkraut)
- Fish
- Fish sauce
- Fruit (bananas, grapes, citrus, pineapple, strawberries)
- Kefir (including coconut)
- Mushrooms
- Pork
- Shellfish
- Smoked fish
- Smoked meat
- Spinach
- Vinegar
- Yogurt (including coconut milk varieties)

heart, anxiety, nausea, and vomiting. Histamine intolerance can be caused by genetic predisposition (like a mutation in the enzymes that degrade histamine or methylation), or more commonly, an overgrowth of bacteria in the gut (like SIBO, see page 84). Sometimes, histamine intolerance can be improved by treating the underlying root cause. Talk to your key player about testing and treatment.

Histamine content in food is a direct product of how it has been handled and processed. Meat, fish, and shellfish naturally produce histamine as soon as they are butchered or harvested, and this histamine level increases as time goes on. Cured or aged meats, as well as foods that have been improperly handled or stored, will have a higher histamine content than fresh. During the fermentation process, histamine is created by the multiplying bacteria.

If you find that you are reacting to foods high in histamine, following a low-histamine diet can help manage symptoms. Histamine intolerance is not like an allergy, where a very small amount of a substance can cause a problem, but more like a threshold that is passed before symptoms appear. You may find that you react to some high-histamine foods but not others, or you may get comfortable with serving sizes and combinations that allow you to stay below your personal threshold. In addition, it is important to work with your key player on pinpointing the root cause of your histamine intolerance, as it can sometimes be resolved.

Dysbiosis

It is common for those with autoimmune disease to suffer from an imbalance of gut microflora, otherwise known as dysbiosis. This can present itself in a multitude of ways—maybe you simply have too few of the beneficial bacteria that are necessary for regulating the immune system, making essential vitamins, and keeping your colon healthy. Others may have bacterial infections, overgrowths, or issues with yeast and parasites. Many imbalances in gut flora lead to other imbalances, and you can be left with a complex web of gut problems that is difficult to unravel.

A big red flag that you may be suffering from dysbiosis is an intolerance to carbohydrates, even when contained in a "real food" package like fruit or tubers such as sweet potatoes. Often, these foods contain the "food" that these organisms thrive on, causing symptoms to worsen. Although avoidance of carbohydrates can be helpful for managing symptoms, it is not a great long-term approach because you end up also starving your beneficial flora, which can have negative conse-

quences. If you notice you don't tolerate certain carbohydrates or continue to have digestive symptoms after 30 to 90 days in the elimination phase, it would be wise to ask your key player for a comprehensive stool test, one that can help diagnose your issue.

Treatment of dysbiosis can be multiphase and generally takes time. First, it may be necessary to kill off the worst offenders with conventional or natural antimicrobial agents. Next, beneficial strains of flora must be slowly reintroduced, and dietary modifications may be necessary to starve out certain species or feed others. The treatment for some types of dysbiosis may be exactly what exacerbates another type, so it is important to work with a practitioner who is using testing to determine the type of treatment required.

DYSBIOSIS CHECKLIST

This is a checklist that will help you determine if you should talk to your key player about being evaluated for dysbiosis.

☐ I have a history of excessive antibiotic use.

☐ I have a history of eating a high-carb diet.

☐ I suffer from constipation or diarrhea.

☐ I suffer from brain fog.

☐ I suffer from abdominal pain, bloating, or gas.

☐ I have foul-smelling stools and/or gas.

☐ I notice my symptoms worsen when I eat sweet foods.

☐ I notice my symptoms worsen when I eat starchy foods.

☐ I crave sweet or starchy foods.

☐ I continue to have skin problems like acne or rashes.

☐ I feel worse in damp or musty environments.

☐ I suffer from frequent headaches.

DIGESTIVE ISSUES

Optimal digestion is necessary to see the benefits of a great diet. Unfortunately, digestive issues can be a common roadblock to success during the elimination phase, as just changing which foods you eat may not be enough to restore optimal gut health. While many of these issues can be remedied by supplements and rarely warrant medical intervention, it may be helpful to have a practitioner guide you to ensure that you are only supplementing in areas where there is a clear need.

Common Digestive Issues

- **LOW STOMACH ACID (HYPOCHLORHYDRIA)—** We need adequate stomach acid to fully break down and digest proteins and prepare our bodies for further digestion. If you are experiencing acid reflux, indigestion, or noticing large pieces of food in your stool, ask your key player to determine if you have enough stomach acid.

- **BILE INSUFFICIENCY—**Bile is necessary to emulsify and digest the healthy fats that we eat. Not having enough bile can lead to symptoms like nausea, pain, diarrhea, and greasy or fatty stools. Those experiencing these issues, as well as those without gall-bladders, should ask their key player for support in this area.

- **ENZYME DEFICIENCY—**Your pancreas makes enzymes that are essential for the complete breakdown of proteins, fats, and carbohydrates in your diet. Lacking enzymes can lead to incomplete digestion and gastrointestinal distress.

- **LACK OF BENEFICIAL GUT FLORA—**Beneficial flora, otherwise known as probiotics, are an essential and necessary component of healthy gut function. If you have a history of antibiotic use (which can wipe out the bad *and* the good) or are experiencing digestive issues, you may not have enough beneficial bacteria in your gut. Three common types of probiotics are *Lactobacillus* species, *Bifidobacterium* species, and soil-based probiotics (various species found in the soil).

OTHER ISSUES
Additional Food Allergies

Although the Autoimmune Protocol removes most foods likely to be problematic for you from an autoimmune standpoint, it can be common for you to have additional food allergies and/or sensitivities to foods on the "include" list. If you notice that you are getting new or worsening symptoms after introducing a food you typically did not eat before, or now are eating much more frequently, it is important to remove that food as a potential allergen. This often happens with foods like coconut, which is pretty uncommon in the modern diet but can be heavily relied upon as a dairy replacement in the elimination phase. It is important to also exclude any food you have a known allergy, sensitivity, or intolerance to while on the Autoimmune Protocol.

Not Enough Carbohydrates

If you find yourself unusually tired while on the elimination phase, you may have inadvertently started eating a low-carbohydrate diet. While the Autoimmune Protocol is not by definition low-carb, you can end up here especially if you don't go out of your way to eat compliant starchy carbs. If you are having issues, the fix is simple—try to include some starchy carbs in your diet on a daily basis. Everyone has a unique individual tolerance to the amount of carbohydrate in his or her diet so we don't have a specific recommendation, but it is worth trying to up your intake if you find yourself feeling run down and fatigued.

Elimination-Diet-Friendly Starchy Carbohydrates

- Arrowroot
- Cassava
- Parsnips
- Plantains
- Sweet potatoes
- Tapioca
- Taro
- Turnips
- Winter squash (like pumpkin or butternut squash)
- Yams

CALL TO ACTION

This chapter is extensive and dense with information. It's with good reason though; nourishing yourself is the basis of living well with autoimmune disease. The foundation for success is laid by how you choose to fuel your body. Pouring the wrong kind of fuel into the gas tank of a car destroys it, ruining each part of its carefully assembled machinery. This is a very apt metaphor for your body; exactly the same principles apply.

We've worked to show you that taking the time to learn about sound nutritional choices and then putting them into practice with planning, preparation, and balance will pay huge dividends. After you've decided on the right dietary transition for yourself, dive in and give your body time to receive the benefits of increased nourishment. If you find yourself with lingering issues even after making major dietary change, don't be discouraged. Simply troubleshoot, with the help of your health-care team, to get to the root causes of your symptoms.

This point on the journey is likely to be one of the, if not *the most*, transformative experiences. Learning to *nourish* your unique system is a delicate and demanding process, but the wisdom gained is likely to change your life.

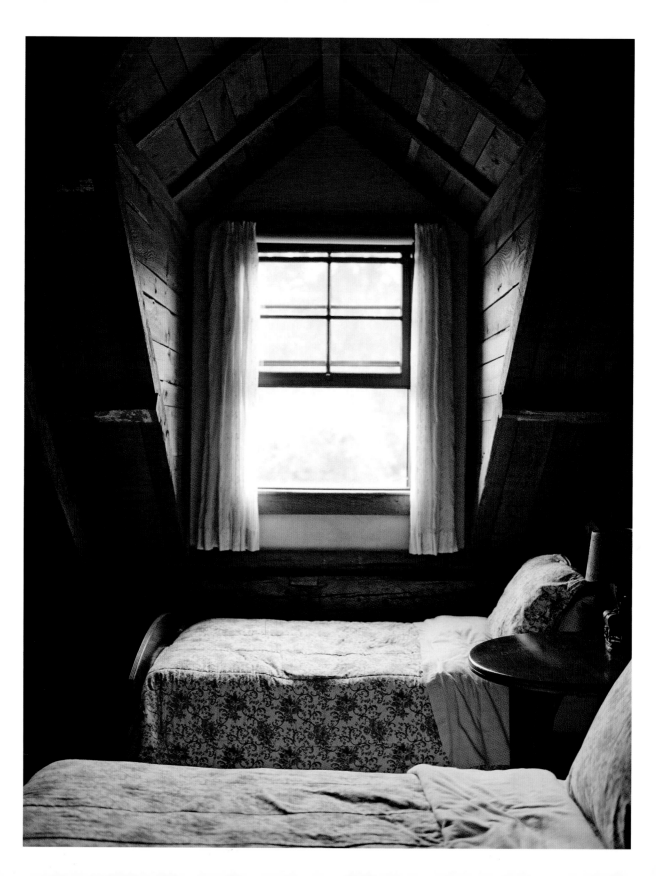

CHAPTER 4

Rest

"Improving the quality, duration, and timing of your sleep is one of the single most powerful interventions you can make to improve your health." —CHRIS KRESSER, *YOUR PERSONAL PALEO CODE*

THE EVALUATION AND IMPROVEMENT OF YOUR sleep is a meaningful and necessary step in managing your chronic illness. Chris Kresser says it perfectly—sleep is not optional. If you have trouble falling asleep, staying asleep, are tired upon waking, or feel sleepy or fatigued throughout your day, it is clear you are in deep need of implementing some better sleep hygiene and/or troubleshooting your barriers to sleep. Sleep problems are prevalent in our culture, and what most people consider normal sleep is anything but. It is safe to assume that *everyone* has steps to take in improving his or her sleep. Excess inflammation, less cellular regeneration and repair, lowered immunity, and imbalanced hormones can be the outcome of too little rest. Even if you have addressed dietary issues and made other lifestyle changes, they won't be effective if you aren't sleeping properly. In this chapter, we'll be covering the basics of sleep as well as giving you some practical tips to integrate into your healing routine.

WHAT IS SLEEP?

Despite the fact that everyone sleeps to some degree or another every night, the exact reasons why you sleep, as well as what exactly happens while you sleep, largely remain a mystery. While sleep was originally thought of as a dormant, inactive state, it is becoming increasingly understood that your body is active during sleep, with many important functions occurring *only* when you are sleeping. Research is getting closer to unraveling this mystery, but for now, most of what we know is that good physical and mental health are deeply dependent on the processes that take place while you are in this restful state.

Sleep is triggered by a mix of neurotransmitters (hormonal messengers in the brain) and hormones, as well as increased sleep pressure, which builds as you are awake and culminates as you ready yourself to fall asleep. Falling asleep takes you gradually from a conscious to an unconscious state. Once you are asleep, your body progresses in and out of five stages, in a cyclical fashion. If your body achieves the adequate duration and timing of all of the stages, without interruption, giving it a chance to perform all of those functions necessary for optimal health, you wake up feeling energized and refreshed. Unfortunately, this is often harder to achieve than it should be. Sleep deprivation causes negative consequences in our health on a regular basis.

A GROWING PROBLEM

The lack of sleep our culture is experiencing has reached epidemic status. While we need 7 to 8 hours per night, 35 percent of adults report getting less than 6 hours of sleep. Fifty years ago, that figure was 2 percent. Why is this so? A couple of factors—as time goes on, our culture continues to glorify productivity and workaholism more than restoration and relaxation. Time spent sleeping has steadily decreased as time spent working has increased. In addition, exposure to light (especially "blue light" emitted by TV screens, computers, and smartphones) after the sun has gone down deeply impacts our body's own natural rhythms. This technology has enabled us to work round-the-clock and override the natural process that

causes us to sleep. As troubling as it is, sleeplessness has become the norm and a culturally accepted part of modern life, with most of us unaware of its consequences.

While the majority of people simply don't get enough quantity or quality of sleep, sleep disorders and other issues are widespread and growing. Nearly 1 in 4 Americans suffer from sleep disorders that are in turn linked to health issues like depression, obesity, type 2 diabetes, cardiovascular disease, and overall risk of death. These disorders include:

- Insomnia—the inability to sleep

- Sleep apnea—interrupted breathing during sleep

- Narcolepsy—the inability to control the sleep-wake cycle

While there are treatments for these conditions, they only help manage symptoms and do not attempt to fix the underlying imbalance.

One thing is clear—the rising prevalence of sleep issues combined with the ongoing cultural shift that devalues the need for sleep is not good for our health. Despite a growing epidemic of enormous proportion, most people live unaware of the consequences of sleep deprivation, such as:

- Decreased immunity (such as catching a cold or flu more easily)

- Decreased stress tolerance

- Propensity for weight gain, obesity, and diabetes

- Reduced learning capacity
- Greater risk for chronic disease
- Increased fatigue and lowered productivity
- Mental health issues
- Systemic inflammation
- Increased risk of death

Clearly, the effects on our health are detrimental and we need to reprioritize this forgotten area of our lives. Taking care of our sleep would put a huge dent in the vast modern disease burden we have today, as well as actually making us level-headed and efficient!

HOW DOES SLEEP WORK?

In order to describe some of the things that can go wrong with sleep, we must first address what we know about the factors that control our sleep and wake cycles. What we know about these cycles today was developed as the two-process model of sleep regulation proposed by Swiss sleep researcher Alexander Borbély, MD. Another sleep researcher, Dan Pardi, MS, developed terminology to describe this model, with two opposing factors affecting these cycles. The first is sleep pressure, which is the increasing need to sleep that starts when you wake up and accumulates the longer you go without sleep. As sleep pressure builds, you become more tired until you are able to fall asleep. The second is wake drive, which produces alertness and wakefulness in contrast to sleep pressure. During the day, your wake drive increases and keeps you alert and your energy levels stable. Unlike sleep pressure, which is regulated by the time that has passed since sleeping last, wake drive is driven by your circadian rhythm, which is a 24-hour cycle, and naturally dissipates when it is time to sleep.

This is a delicate system that can be disrupted in many ways. For instance, by not getting enough sleep one night, you are left with sleep debt, which will then be tacked on to the next time you sleep. Even if that next sleep cycle is optimal, you may still wake up feeling unrested because you did not sleep enough to cancel out the additional sleep debt. A common practice is to get less sleep during the workweek and then make up for it on the weekend, but it is rarely possible to achieve without leaving some outstanding debt week after week. This leads to a chronic "negative balance" and long-term impacts. Anyone who has been through an exam week in college knows firsthand how sleep debt can catch up with you!

Your circadian rhythm is a 24-hour cycle of biological processes that has an intricate relationship with your sleep-wake cycle. Your brain is in control of these processes, which are carried out through the release of hormones that rise and fall, depending on the time of day. Some hormones, like cortisol, increase in the morning as you wake up and provide the energy you need to get through the day. In contrast, melatonin increases a couple hours before bed and promotes drowsiness to induce sleep. There are many factors that

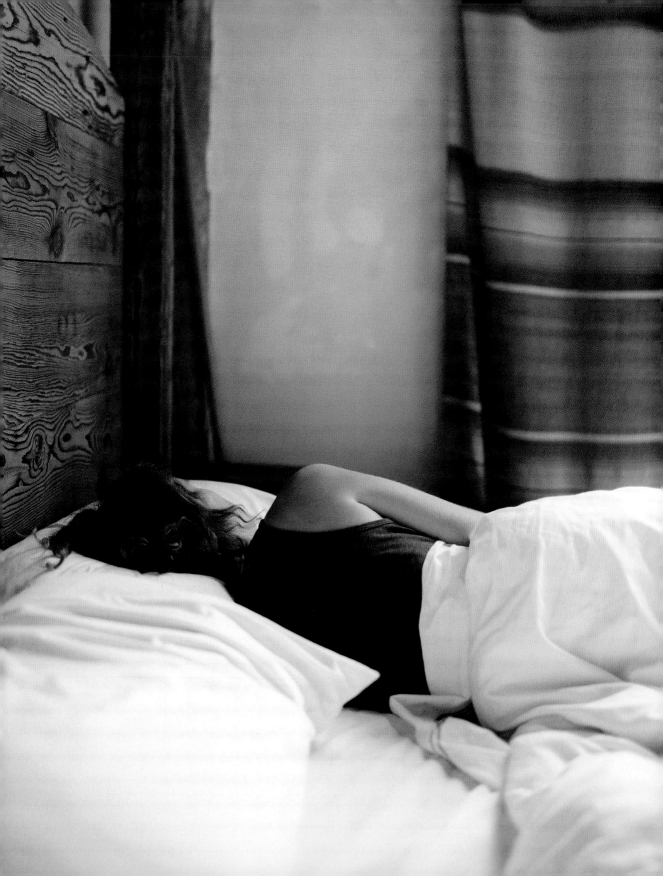

impact your circadian rhythm, but one of the most powerful is the light-dark cycle. Exposure to bright light (especially daylight) during the daytime and complete darkness at night helps our body regulate this cycle. There are many factors that can disrupt your circadian rhythm, which can cause sleepiness during the day and wakefulness at night. We'll be discussing these later on in the chapter.

SLEEP AND HEALING

How does sleep fit in with the healing process? Getting the appropriate quality and duration of sleep is absolutely necessary for healing and recovery. "Dialing in" your sleep can lower inflammation, regulate and strengthen the immune system, and positively impact hunger hormones and metabolism. Your body engages in the restorative process of tissue repair and regeneration only when you are sleeping—which means if an autoimmune disease is taking its toll, it should be important to you! In addition, adequate sleep enhances memory and mental clarity, improves energy levels, helps manage stress, and keeps you happy. While it may not be the most obvious step in your healing journey, it is an absolutely essential one!

HOW MUCH SLEEP DO YOU NEED?

Sleep needs are highly individual, but research shows that most adults need 7 to 8 hours of uninterrupted sleep. You may feel that you function just fine on the national average of 6 hours; if you notice a pattern of feeling excessively tired in the morning, possibly needing stimulants such

as caffeine, and/or having more energy at night, it is a sign that your sleep needs are not being met.

On the other hand, you may feel that you need an excessive amount of sleep, perhaps 10 to 12 hours per night, to feel rested. This is not uncommon for those suffering from chronic illness and is often a symptom of autoimmune disease (like Hashimoto's thyroiditis). If it is at all possible, allow yourself to meet your body's needs. Sometimes, as underlying causes are resolved (such as the lack of thyroid hormone with Hashimoto's) or sleep quality improves due to lifestyle changes (see the lifestyle guide on page 243), you may find yourself feeling refreshed and needing less sleep.

As it applies to healing, it is important to err on the side of too much sleep rather than too little. As we have outlined in this chapter, sleep is absolutely essential to the deep healing and tissue repair necessary for living well with autoimmune disease. Do yourself a favor and make sure to get in bed with plenty of time to spare, and give yourself that extra hour or two to sleep in in the morning. Your body will thank you!

For those who regularly wake up with an alarm and may be unaware of their body's natural sleep needs, we have designed a sleep exploration exercise on page 110 to help you determine your requirements.

WHAT INFLUENCES A GOOD NIGHT'S SLEEP?

There are many issues that can factor into sleep disturbances: diet, stress, circadian rhythm disruption, environmental influences, and our health conditions themselves are just a few that we'll be focusing on here. Understanding how each of these impacts both sleep quantity and quality can be useful in trying to combat the negative effects.

Diet

Although it may not be readily apparent, our diets can have an immense impact on our sleep. Understanding the basic reasons why can help you make the connections and hopefully allow you to institute a few simple changes.

Caffeine consumption (whether coffee, tea, or chocolate) can be a dietary factor in sleep disturbances. This is because caffeine stimulates the production of cortisol (there's that "wake up" hormone again!). These levels can stay elevated for 6 hours or more after the caffeine is consumed. Some people find that even 1 cup of coffee or tea in the morning (or even chocolate, for the very sensitive) impacts their sleep the following night. You may feel like, over time, you are more and more tolerant to caffeine, with it affecting you less and less. This is partly true, but complete tolerance never occurs, so thinking that it doesn't affect you is simply wrong.

Alcohol consumption can be another dietary factor in sleep disturbances, for a few reasons. Alcohol is a diuretic, which means it forces the body to excrete water and can lead to dehydration. If you've ever drunk too much and then found yourself awake in the middle of the night needing a big glass of water, you understand this effect. Alcohol consumption can also trigger the release of insulin, while simultaneously impairing the rectifying release of glucose from the liver to prevent a too-low blood sugar. Although many people think a nightcap helps them sleep well, both alcohol-related dehydration and blood sugar crashes disrupt sleep.

Both low-fat and low-carb diets get it wrong when it comes to sleeping well. These dietary approaches can lead to poor sleep, even insomnia. We all know the feeling of being just a bit too hungry when we hit the pillow—trying to maintain a fast of 7 to 9 hours with a hungry tummy is simply unrealistic and instead results in tossing and turning. In addition, research shows that dense carbohydrate sources, like starchy vegetables, also help us sleep better. Carbs help the amino acid tryptophan enter the pineal gland, deep in the center of the brain, where it contributes to the production of melatonin (that sleep hormone). Carbs also help prevent your blood sugar from dropping overnight. When blood sugar gets too low, the hormone cortisol is released (that alertness hormone). If you consistently wake up suddenly, feeling a bit anxious between 2 a.m. and 4 a.m., it's probably a blood sugar crash from eating too little carbohydrate at your evening meal.

Finally, there is the issue of food sensitivities. Reactions caused by a food you are sensitive to can vary wildly, and one of the possible responses could be trouble sleeping. You may find that trouble falling asleep, staying asleep, or just plain feeling unrested is the result of consuming a particular food. Be aware of this possible reaction either improving as you eliminate foods or coming back as you experiment with food reintroductions.

Chronic Stress

Most of us understand, intuitively, that chronic stress contributes to sleep disturbances. That awful, pressure-cooker job is hard to stop thinking about, even when it's time to hit the pillow, or maybe the arguments you've been having with your partner leave you feeling angry and amped for hours each night. What exactly is causing that sleeplessness in response to stress?

You guessed it—it's cortisol again! Chronic stress stimulates constant production of cortisol, which causes imbalances in your hormonal cycle and disrupts your circadian rhythms. Cortisol needs to steadily decrease during the day and allow melatonin to pick up in the evening. When it stays elevated, your body doesn't receive the signal to turn off and rest. You may fall asleep, but if your hormonal balance is off, the natural sleep cycle can be disrupted, leading to poor-quality sleep. To make matters worse, lack of sleep is itself a form of chronic stress, making the cycle a worsening loop. Actively managing stress, especially that long-term kind, is extremely important to healthy sleep.

Circadian Rhythm Disruption

Circadian rhythm refers to your "body clock." Humans (and animals, plants, and even microbes) go through specific biological processes at key points in a roughly 24-hour cycle. This rhythm is most influenced by alternating periods of sunlight and darkness, known as the light-dark cycle.

There are stages in life where the rhythm goes through some changes, despite these light-dark signals. As infants, our clocks are not mature and do not respond as readily to light-dark signals. Then, as teens, we typically experience sleep phase delay, where we feel alert later into the night and want to stay asleep later into the day. Finally, in our old age, we may experience another shift referred to as advanced sleep phase syndrome, where we feel tired earlier in the day and become alert in the very early morning hours. Anyone who has ever cared for an infant who is waking every few hours during the night or parented a teen who is up listening to music and laughing with friends at midnight can attest to the fact that regardless of these recognized rhythm shifts over our life spans, doing everything possible to promote the regularity of our body clocks is hugely important.

You've already heard about cortisol and melatonin, the two key hormones affecting sleep. These hormones help keep the timing of the circadian rhythm steady. Cortisol increases in the few hours before we wake up and is at its highest early in the day. Melatonin increases in the few hours before we go to bed and is at its highest in the wee

(continued on page 102)

WHERE ARE YOU ON THE SLEEP-QUALITY SPECTRUM?

This test will help you determine if your sleep quality is optimal or needs work. Give yourself a point for every item on the list that applies to you, and then total your score and see whether improving your sleep should be a priority.

____ My energy is not stable throughout the day.

____ I am dependent on waking up with an alarm.

____ I feel rushed to get to bed at night.

____ I have trouble falling asleep.

____ I wake more than once during the night.

____ I often wake up before my alarm and am unable to fall back asleep.

____ I have trouble concentrating.

____ I have been told that I snore.

____ I have been told I toss and turn at night.

____ I grind my teeth at night.

____ I find myself unable to fall asleep because I am worrying about things.

____ I lie awake for a long time before falling asleep.

____ I have trouble waking up.

____ I need caffeine in the morning to get me going.

____ I wake up out of breath and/or I have been told I hold my breath while I sleep.

____ I wake up sweating.

____ I wake up suddenly with a strong sense of anxiety.

____ I wake up suddenly and feel hunger.

____ Chronic pain prevents me from falling/staying asleep.

____ I am sleepy during the day.

____ I find myself irritable or unable to tolerate stress.

____ I often have a hard time remembering things.

____ I can't get through the day without a nap.

____ I find myself dozing off during the day, while working and/or driving.

____ I feel like I am in a daze or brain fog.

1—9 LOW PRIORITY—Good job! Your sleep quality is most likely good enough for optimal health and healing. We suggest looking over some of the recommendations in the following chapters, as you may have other areas (such as diet, stress management, movement, or connection) that take a higher priority in your healing journey.

10—14 MODERATE PRIORITY—Looks like your sleep could use some work! Time to dig into the recommendations that follow in this chapter to see if you can make some improvements. Your sleep is not as poor as it could be, but now is the time to act before things get worse.

15—HIGH PRIORITY—Uh-oh! It appears that your sleep quality is extremely low. This is a strong indicator that you need to prioritize and focus on the recommendations laid out in this chapter. In addition, you may want to talk to your key player to help you unravel some of the underlying factors that are impacting your sleep.

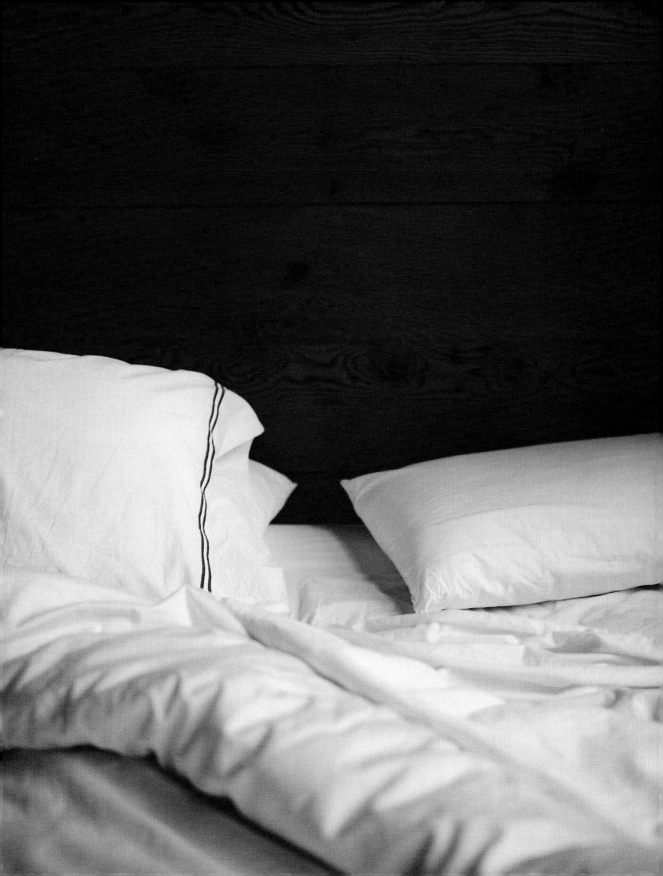

hours of the morning. Production of this hormone ramps up with darkness and diminishes with light exposure. If the production of either cortisol or melatonin is disturbed, we soon find our sleep is a mess. Sooner or later, this also means we are more susceptible to illness and disease, since both hormones are major players in immune regulation. Protecting our circadian rhythms helps reinforce the balance necessary to live well with autoimmune disease.

Environmental Factors

Sometimes sleep disturbance is about environmental factors, like artificial light, electronics usage, temperature, and noise. We have to obey the laws of nature when it comes to sleep. Sleep is best matched to a particular environment we lived in harmony with for most our existence as a species: dark, free of electronics, cool, and quiet.

We need to minimize exposure to artificial light in the hours before bed and then aim for complete darkness during sleep, otherwise our melatonin production is disrupted. What you may not realize is that this is not just about your eyes, it is also about light exposure to your skin! Your skin is also photosensitive, so paying attention to this environmental factor can have a big impact on your sleep.

The use of electronics, in general, as well as electronics in our bedrooms, disrupts sleep. The blue-spectrum light being emitted from your TV, laptop, tablet, or cell phone is particularly disruptive to melatonin production. Removing them from your bedroom eliminates this environmental factor. Disruption isn't only about the light exposure; scrolling through upsetting headlines or having a text chat with friends is not creating the best atmosphere for sleep. Having an emotional buffer between your regular daytime routine and bedtime is important.

Have you ever woken up sweating, only to realize the air-conditioning went out during the night, and the temperature slowly rose in the bedroom until you were so uncomfortable it disrupted your sleep? We need a comfortable but cool overnight temperature in our bedrooms for the best rest. Throughout the day, your body temperature rises and falls in a pattern that is tied to the sleep-wake cycle. Your temperature goes down as bedtime approaches and gets to its lowest point in the very early morning hours. After that, it starts to go up again. A bedroom that is too hot can affect your body's natural temperature controls and result in poor sleep. Sleep researchers have found that a temperature around 65°F is about right.

Noise is the final environmental factor we are exploring here and probably the most obvious. Anything from children, pets, electronic notifications, neighbors, to street noise can disrupt your sleep. It goes without saying, but a quiet room is best.

Health Conditions

For some, sleep disturbances may be the result of autoimmune or related diseases.

For example, pain from your rheumatoid arthritis or the various symptoms of your other diseases can ruin a good night's sleep. Immune cells that play a role in your disease might also be to blame, as they secrete a range of hormones that disrupt the circadian rhythm. In this case, much like with chronic stress, a negative cycle can develop where the autoimmune disease is causing lack of sleep and lack of sleep is worsening the disease.

TROUBLESHOOTING SLEEP

You know you need to work on your sleep—but where do you start? There are many areas where small adjustments can yield big results. Here, we cover those areas that can be refined for better quality and duration of sleep. Take note of anything that rings true for you, and use the "Troubleshooting Checklist" on page 109 to incorporate these recommendations into your routine.

Diet

There are a few dietary interventions that may have a positive impact on sleep. The first is to eliminate or reduce caffeine from your diet. You will want to make a plan depending on where you are on the spectrum of caffeine intake (quitting cold-turkey is not advised!). If you are someone who relies on a few cups of coffee a day to keep you going, and *especially* if you get headaches or feel groggy without your morning cup, work on weaning yourself gradually off the caffeine. You can either blend in some decaffeinated coffee (Swiss Water Process

coffee has fewer chemicals) starting with 25 percent and increasing the percentage, or start drinking less total volume on a week-to-week basis. Some coffee drinkers have an easier time transitioning to black tea, and then green tea, which both progressively have less caffeine. If you are a tea drinker, you may be surprised to find out how much caffeine is in your black and green tea! Chocolate can also be a problem for those who are very sensitive. If you are having trouble sleeping, it is good to wean off all caffeine (even chocolate!) for a month to see if that is the source of your problem. When you go to add it back, you may find that you have a threshold of tolerance or a cutoff for time of day where it affects your sleep. A common example might be that you tolerate 1 cup of coffee in the morning, but if you have any more than that, or any in the afternoon, it impacts your sleep.

On the other hand are depressants, which can have an equally negative impact. Alcohol can be a major factor for some people, and while it can feel like it helps you fall asleep, it is likely to prevent you from staying asleep because of its effects on hydration and blood sugar, as mentioned above. Similar to caffeine, it is helpful to avoid all alcohol for a month or more to determine how it affects your sleep.

The next dietary intervention that may help your sleep is adjusting your carb intake at dinnertime or before bed. Starchy carbohydrates (like sweet potatoes, yams, plantains, and winter squash, if you are in the elimination phase), especially when combined with a high-quality fat (olive oil, coconut oil, or pastured lard or tallow) help keep you satiated throughout the night. Most people sleep best when their stomach is neither too full nor too empty, and having a few-hours' window between dinner and bedtime is optimal. This changes if you are specifically suffering from issues with blood-sugar regulation and find that you wake up a few hours after going to sleep—

ANGIE'S EXPERIENCE

When I was my sickest, sleep was a major issue for me. Despite crushing fatigue, I had a very hard time falling and staying asleep. The staying asleep part was particularly awful! I woke up almost every night between 2 and 4 a.m. in a terrifying panic. I was often sweating profusely, my heart was beating rapidly, and I would lie there sure I was experiencing my final moments. Diet was playing a huge role in this problem— my blood sugar was crashing each night, causing my adrenal glands to kick into high gear. That surge of cortisol was what had me waking up constantly in terror. To make matters worse, I was compounding the problem by attempting to use alcohol to help me sleep. I thought that a nightly glass of wine might help me rest, but, in fact, it was exacerbating the blood-sugar crash and severely dehydrating me. When I began to include more carbohydrate and fat into my evening meal, and quit alcohol altogether for a long period, my sleep improved immensely. If I focus on diet aimed at well-balanced blood sugar and keep alcohol consumption to special occasions, I'm almost guaranteed a restful night.

here you can try having a small balanced snack with some starchy carbohydrate, fat, and protein just before bed. Everyone should avoid sweet or sugary foods in the evening or before bed, as they are likely to spike blood sugar and cause a midnight crash, waking you up! It may take some experimenting to figure out what works best for you, but adjustments here can have an impact on quality of sleep.

Last, food allergies and sensitivities can absolutely impact sleep. If you haven't done an elimination and reintroduction protocol, review the details in Chapter 3 for guidance on pinpointing those trouble foods. You may find that your sleep improves after eliminating particular foods from your diet.

Stress Management

If you are concerned about your sleep, stress management needs to be a part of your routine. Start a mindfulness practice and make sure you follow through with it. This could be as simple as taking 1 or more 5-minute breaks during the day to sit still, be quiet, and listen to your breath. You may have other activities that help you manage your stress effectively— meditation, hiking, yoga, walking, taking a bath, getting a massage, or just being in nature. Whatever you find relaxing and restorative, make an effort to include that in your daily routine to see how it impacts your sleep. If you need more help in this area, we'll be addressing it in depth in Chapter 5.

SUPPORTING YOUR NATURAL RHYTHMS

As you found out earlier in this chapter, it is very easy for your natural circadian rhythm to get offtrack from exposure to light at the wrong times during the day. This fix goes a little against cultural norms, but can be incredibly effective at promoting quality sleep. First, you will want to make sure to time your sleep-wake cycle as close as possible to sunset and sunrise. For most of us, this means going to bed earlier and waking up earlier. Being in bed by 10 and up by 7 is a great goal. It may take some prioritizing and rearranging to

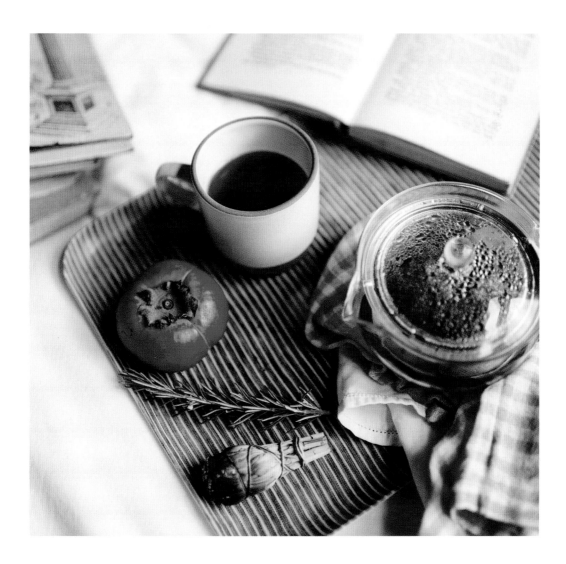

make sure you are ready to wind down at the appropriate time, but you will make up for it with increased energy and productivity after improving your sleep.

Next, you want to make sure to minimize your exposure to blue-spectrum light after the sun goes down. This can mean dimming the lights, installing blue-light-blocking software on your computer and devices, or wearing blue-light-blocking glasses in the evenings (see Resources on page 261). You also want to make sure that your bedroom is completely dark and free from light pollution (you may want to invest in some blackout shades). Don't underestimate this recommendation! Minimizing your exposure to blue light before bed and all light at night helps your body make the hormones necessary for initiating and staying asleep.

Similarly, you want to *expose* yourself to blue light during the earlier part of the day, preferably in the morning right after waking up. This helps your body make the hormones that wake you up and get you going for the day. If you can get outside for at least 20 minutes without sunglasses and let nature work its magic on resetting your internal clock, that is the best way to go! For those who can't make it outside, a blue-light therapy lamp can be a good compromise (see Resources on page 261).

A note about shift work—we know that for some people, their job makes it nearly impossible to sleep and rise with the sun. If you need to work during the night, you need to be even more diligent about protecting your circadian rhythms and stay-

ing on a regular cycle. You can simulate a 24-hour light-and-dark cycle with the use of blue-light-blocking glasses, a very dark sleeping area, as well as a blue-light-emitting lamp.

Practice Good Sleep Hygiene

It is important to have a regular bedtime routine that is conducive to helping you fall asleep. Going straight from work, exercise, an intense TV show, or a heated discussion with a loved one to immediately trying to fall asleep does not set you up to achieve that goal. Try to plan a relaxing activity or ritual to repeat every night before you go to bed. This might be something as simple as washing your face and doing a short meditation, reading a book (careful with novels that are too intense or stimulating!), taking a bath with epsom salts, or journaling. Avoid watching TV, working, having tense discussions, doing strenuous exercise, paying bills, scrolling social media, or anything else that is going to prevent you from relaxing and falling asleep.

Equally important is making sure your sleep environment is comfortable and conducive to sleep. Your bed should be clean and cozy and your room cool and dark. If there is too much light coming in through your windows, consider investing in blackout shades, and make sure to cover up any blinking or solid lights from electronic devices with dark tape (or better yet—get them out of the bedroom!). If you can't control the light situation, you may want to purchase an eye mask. If noise is an issue, you may want a device to make white noise (an air purifier or fan helps here) or to use earplugs.

If you can, get all technology out of the bedroom and don't use that space for working or watching television. Charge devices outside the bedroom, and make sure they are set not to ding, buzz, or beep during sleeping hours (for those of you who are worried about emergencies, you can set many devices to ring on second call or have a select few numbers who can always reach you). Some of these recommendations are among the most difficult to implement, because poor sleep hygiene is ingrained in our culture. As you start to make sleep more of a priority, these steps will come more naturally (see the lifestyle guide on page 243)!

Movement

Getting more exercise during the day can help you fall asleep easier as well as improve the quality of your sleep. If you are having trouble with your sleep and don't get much exercise, try starting a gentle exercise like walking or yoga. If you do well with more intense exercise, you can try running, cycling, lifting weights, or anything else that you find pleasurable that is also not too energy-depleting—just don't do these activities in the few hours before bed! We'll be talking more about optimal exercise in Chapter 6.

Supplementation

You'll need guidance from your health-care team here, but there are some supplements that can be helpful for troubleshooting issues with sleep, like magnesium, various herbal preparations, and other nutrients. Most people find that taking magnesium before bed helps them relax and fall asleep more easily. We don't recommend melatonin unless prescribed by a doctor because it can cause the body to make less of this essential hormone. There are other herbs and nutrients that can be helpful for balancing sleep. If you've worked through some of the previous recommendations and are still having trouble, it might be time to ask your key player or support player to assist you with putting together a protocol.

Naps

If you are unable to get quality, uninterrupted sleep during the night, napping might be necessary for you. For a lot of people, napping can be a problem because it lessens sleep pressure and makes it more difficult to fall asleep at night. If you feel like you don't get sleepy enough before bed and have a hard time falling asleep, naps are likely to exacerbate this problem. That being said, if your sleep is being interrupted for other reasons, such as chronic pain, a new baby, or otherwise, naps may be necessary for you to meet your body's requirement for sleep.

For those who are lacking an hour or two of quality sleep per night, napping isn't a replacement for that sleep—be sure to follow all of the recommendations above before resorting to regular naps to make up the difference. In general, a

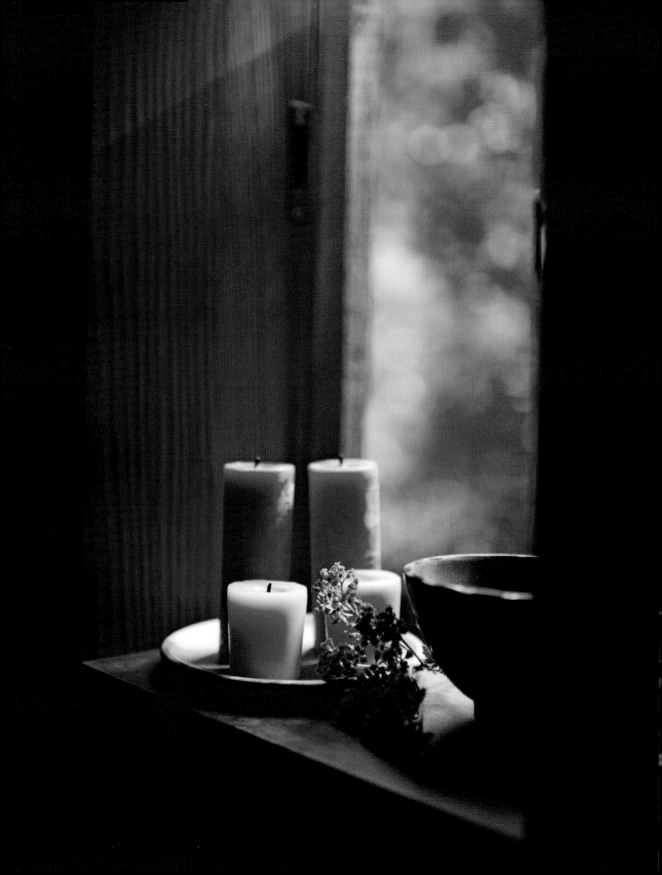

TROUBLESHOOTING CHECKLIST

Use this checklist to determine if you have ticked all of the boxes as you troubleshoot some of the underlying causes of sleep issues. If you are still struggling and find some of these unchecked, it's time to dig in and explore these areas!

☐ I've eliminated or reduced caffeine from my diet for at least 30 days.

☐ I avoid drinking alcohol before bed.

☐ I include starchy carbohydrates and healthy fats in my diet at dinnertime.

☐ I avoid sugar or sweet foods in the evening, especially before bed.

☐ I've done an elimination diet to explore the possibility of food allergies and/or sensitivities.

☐ I incorporate stress-management activities (mindfulness practices, meditation, walking, yoga, massage, or breathwork) into my daily routine.

☐ I go to bed early (10 p.m. or earlier) and wake up early, close to the setting and rising of the sun.

☐ I minimize my exposure to blue light after the sun goes down (through the use of blue-light-blocking glasses and software or dimming the lights).

☐ I maximize my exposure to blue light in the morning (either by going outside or using a light-therapy lamp).

☐ I use blackout shades, an eye mask, or other methods to ensure that my bedroom is completely dark when I go to bed.

☐ I have set up my bedroom to be conducive to sleep—comfortable, cool, quiet, and dark. If I cannot control the temperature or noise, I use a fan or earplugs.

☐ I keep all technology out of the bedroom.

☐ I have set my devices not to go off during sleep hours.

☐ I avoid stressful situations and/or work before bed.

☐ I move an appropriate amount throughout the day.

☐ I avoid intense exercise before bed.

☐ I've talked to someone on my health-care team about using magnesium or other supplements before bed to help me relax and fall asleep.

☐ I've ruled out underlying sleep conditions like insomnia, sleep apnea, restless leg syndrome, and narcolepsy with my health-care team.

20- to 30-minute nap is restorative and less likely to interrupt regular sleep. An hour or longer nap feels better for some people, but it is more likely to make it difficult to fall asleep later. You will need to experiment and see what works well for you. Uninterrupted sleep at night is preferable over napping because your body is more easily able to reach the deeper and more restorative stages of sleep. Napping can help make up a deficit—just don't use it as a replacement for getting to bed on time!

If you are someone with chronic sleep disturbances, any sleep should be encouraged, including napping. Sometimes, like when there is a new baby in the family, it is not possible to get uninterrupted sleep. In this case, make an effort to get sleep whenever time will allow.

Ruling Out Underlying Conditions

If you've made a good effort to try all of these troubleshooting points and are still not experiencing success, you will want to talk to your key player about investigating underlying conditions or to see if your sleep issues are due to your already-diagnosed conditions. Conducting a sleep study can be helpful in determining why you may not be getting the quality or duration of sleep you need and can give your practitioner valuable information to help gauge what kind of treatment is necessary for resolution.

Sleep Exploration Exercise

This exercise is to help those who regularly wake up with an alarm determine if they are getting enough sleep. While this exercise won't be as useful for those who have insomnia or trouble staying asleep, if you always wake up with an alarm and struggle to get to bed on time, you may be surprised to find out how much sleep your body actu-

ally craves. Try this exercise over a long weekend or another 3-day stretch where it will be okay for you to potentially oversleep. This information can help you determine an appropriate bedtime that gives you enough sleep to meet your needs.

- Review the checklist on page 109 to make sure that you have all of the basic requirements in place (cool, quiet, dark bedroom free from interruptions).

- For a period of 3 days, make sure you go to bed at the same time, and make sure *not* to set an alarm for the following morning.

- Allow yourself to naturally wake up, calculate how many hours you slept for each night, and then average that.

- This is the amount of sleep you should be aiming for every night.

Bedtime Rituals

Here are some ritual ideas you can get into the habit of including in your bedtime rou-

MICKEY'S EXPERIENCE

I've always had trouble falling asleep, and before prioritizing action in this area, I would lie awake in bed for hours, sometimes 3 to 4 before drifting off into a fitful, restless sleep. Creating and following a bedtime ritual has helped me make progress in this area, and if I follow it, I will fall asleep quickly, stay asleep all night, and wake up feeling refreshed and ready for the day. Two hours before bedtime, I put on amber glasses if I am using a screen and dim the lights in my house, and I prioritize activities that are calming and relaxing (like reading a book, knitting, cuddling with my husband or cat, or gentle stretching). One hour before bedtime, I get things ready for the following day, wash my face and brush my teeth, diffuse some essential oils in the bedroom, and make a cup of tea. Right before I turn out the lights, I enjoy tea while reading or cuddle with my husband. If I am feeling particularly wound up or stressed out, I will do a short meditation or body scan as I fall asleep.

tine to help you relax and get ready for sleep. These activities can act as triggers to get your body and mind into a restful state. Use them alone, or in combinations that work for you.

- Take a hot bath with epsom salts and calming essential oils like lavender.
- Take a few minutes to write in a gratitude journal.
- Engage in a spiritual practice like prayer or meditation.
- Create a "worry list" to help get these items out of your head as you ready for sleep.
- Do some gentle stretching and/or breathwork.
- Dim the lights—you might enjoy candlelight or salt lamps.
- Use aromatherapy or essential oils that are calming or relaxing

- Read a relaxing fictional book (taking care that it isn't too gripping or stimulating).
- Take time to practice your bedtime self-care routine (washing your face, brushing your teeth, moisturizing your skin).
- Listen to calming music.
- Engage in a "body scan"—lying in bed, start at your toes and end at your scalp, tensing each part of your body and releasing it.
- Quietly cuddle or engage in personal contact with your partner or family members.
- Practice a mindfulness routine—focus on your breath, the environment, and body sensations in the moments before sleep.
- Take some time to unplug your devices and place them in another room.
- Prepare your clothes and belongings for the next day.

CALL TO ACTION

Although it is one of our most instinctual biological processes, it can be unusually difficult to "get it right" when it comes to sleep. This is only getting more difficult in our modern world, as research reveals humans are sleeping less and less. A solid understanding of sleep and its importance to healing makes it clear that all the effort is wise—sleep is absolutely necessary to health.

In this chapter, we touched on all the common reasons for sleep disturbances and helped you find ways to address them, as well as ways to assess your unique sleep needs. Every journey requires a few pit stops, moments of refueling and repair, and the autoimmune wellness journey is no exception. Giving priority to *rest* will bring with it many benefits. As writer Thomas Dekker said, "Sleep is that golden chain that binds health and our bodies together."

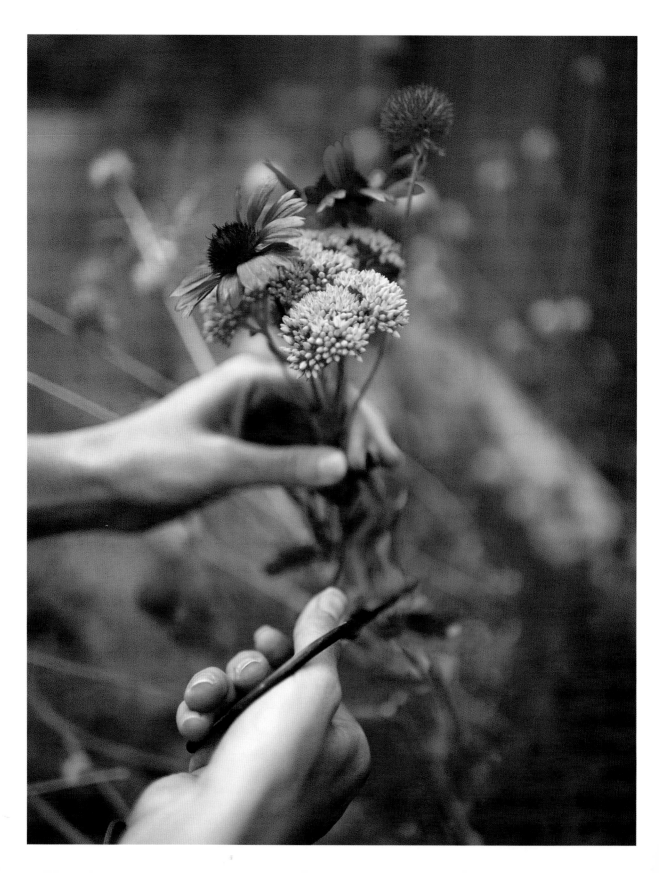

CHAPTER 5

Breathe

"It's not stress that kills us, it's our reaction to it." —DR. HANS SELYE

STRESS IS UBIQUITOUS IN OUR MODERN lives, and we do not value or prioritize the self-care and recovery needed to effectively manage our culture's growing problem. Work and productivity are consistently valued more highly than recovery and vitality, as most of us are expected to work longer hours and with less time off than ever before. Do you frequently feel like you can barely handle the pressures of work and life? You are not alone—a 2014 American Psychological Association report found that 42 percent of Americans say that they are not doing enough to manage their stress levels. In the same report, the most commonly experienced symptoms related to stress were feeling irritable or angry, nervous or anxious, having a lack of interest or motivation, feeling fatigue, feeling overwhelmed, and being depressed. Even considering the sheer volume of people experiencing these symptoms, motivation to make changes is incredibly low, with most continuing on until they physically or mentally cannot cope any longer.

What are we doing to manage this stress? Unfortunately, many people turn to destructive habits like overeating or bingeing on unhealthy foods, skipping meals, drinking alcohol, smoking cigarettes, watching TV, surfing the Internet, or playing video games. If you've ever fallen face-first into a pint of ice cream after experiencing an unexpectedly difficult life event, you understand how stress drives us to these poor lifestyle choices! While stress itself can have long-term negative health consequences, it appears that it also drives us to engage in unhealthy coping habits, compounding the problem.

Whether or not you are aware of the negative consequences of stress on your body, managing it is absolutely essential to improving your health, especially for those suffering from chronic illness. You may be unaware of the fact that underlying health conditions like autoimmune disease are a silent source of stress for your body, making it even more important that you learn to engage in healthy stress-management habits instead of falling into that pint of ice cream. In this chapter, you'll learn about the stress response, common triggers, and how to better practice stress management in your own life.

WHAT IS STRESS?

While the word *stress* usually conjures up a negative response, it is simply a process that helps our bodies adapt to our environments. This can be beneficial, as experiencing and adapting to stress can cause us to become stronger and more able to confront the challenges in our lives. In addition, when we experience an emergency or other appropriately stressful situation, the body is able to rise to the occasion and perform at a higher level in order to avert danger and stay alive. This process developed to help us deal with occasional circumstances where we needed to have better than average ability to perform physically and mentally, such as evading a wild animal attack. In today's world, bears and tigers are uncommon threats to our safety, but situations like a fight with your spouse, an unexpected tax payment, or a traffic ticket on the way to the grocery store can produce the same physiological response. Our bodies respond to stress with a similar cascade of hormones, regardless of the type or source, keeping us in a state of high alert and depleting our energy reserves.

Eustress and Distress

Stress can come in many different forms, from physical, emotional, psychological, or environmental sources, or a combination of these. In addition, stress can be perceived as positive, which is known as eustress, or negative, which is known as distress. Eustress is generally perceived to be within our coping abilities, shorter-term, having beneficial results like better energy or focus, and improving performance. Distress, on the other hand, is stress that is outside our abilities to cope. While it can be short- or long-term, distress is draining and depleting of our energy. In the long run, it contributes to disease and a decrease in performance. It is important to note that what one person may experience as eustress may be distress for another. For instance, moderate exercise feels beneficial to those who are generally healthy. To another person who has an autoimmune condition affecting energy and mobility, exercise can be a cause of distress. In the same vein, if a healthy person were to try to run a marathon without training, his body would be under distress. Whether a stressor has a positive or negative impact has to do with the way that we perceive the stress, as well as our physical ability to handle it.

Stages of the Stress Response

GENERAL ADAPTATION SYNDROME is a model that was originally postulated by stress researcher Dr. Hans Selye to describe the process by which stress affects the body.

Once the body experiences a stressor, there is an initial reaction, followed by movement into further stages depending on the duration of stress, as well as the body's ability to cope. One of the breakthrough facets of this model is that it has a way of showing that there is a limit on the body's ability to handle stress. The three stages of the stress response are as follows:

- **ALARM STAGE**—You have been exposed to a stressor and your body initially reacts to this exposure and activates the "fight-or-flight" response system. The hormones adrenaline and cortisol are released to produce the physical changes that help your body deal with the situation. Heart rate, respiration, and blood pressure increase, and more blood flows to the brain and muscles in order to prepare them for action. Natural anti-inflammatory compounds are released into your body, and your vision, sight, hearing, and awareness all sharpen. Your body is prepared to meet this threat!

- **RESISTANCE STAGE**—You have overcome the stressor, and the threat is either gone or reduced. Your body enters a period of weakness as it uses its remaining energy to recover from the stress response and possible injury or activity. In this stage, your body is still on guard to fight continuing stressors, although without as much strength as it did in the initial reaction.

- **EXHAUSTION STAGE**—You have been fighting stressors for a long period of time and now your body is unable to handle them. At this point, your body won't be able to meet the challenge of any subsequent stressors.

As long as the stress responses you experience are confined to the alarm and resistance stages, your body is able to strengthen and adapt to its circumstances. For instance, starting a new light exercise program is a small stressor to the body. You are unlikely to get "fired up" in the alarm stage the same way as if you were running from a bear, but your body will increase adrenaline and cortisol to meet the demands of the increased movement. As long as you give yourself adequate time in the resistance stage to recover completely, the repeated exercise is likely to strengthen and have a positive impact on your body. In contrast, if you are in poor physical shape and you start an intense exercise program, your alarm stage is going to result in greater stress hormones being produced, as well as more damage and injury to your body. The next time you work out, you are unlikely to be out of the resistance stage, putting your body in the exhaustion stage—unable to handle further stressors, which then leads to additional negative health consequences. Many of us suffering from chronic illness have experienced this very example when starting an exercise routine, which is all the more reason for us to take it easy!

Hormones and Stress

The relationship between three organs in your body, the hypothalamus and pituitary in your brain, and the adrenal glands that sit on top of your kidneys, is called the **HPA (HYPOTHALAMUS-PITUITARY-ADRENAL) AXIS**. This complex system of feedback loops assesses the levels and needs of stress hormones in the body and sets off a chain reaction that ends in the production of these hormones (like cortisol and adrenaline). All it takes to set off this process is the mere *thought* of a stressor, like the presentation deadline at work or a call from your child's school saying she is running a fever. Even if this threat is not physical, your body will continue making stress hormones until it perceives that there are enough to meet the threat and inhibits their production by a negative feedback loop. The hormonal response for different types of stress is the same; it's all about how you perceive the threat!

Understanding the complex mechanics of the HPA axis is not as important as understanding how powerful our thoughts are at driving the response. Some people experience a large amount of physical stress, possibly from a strenuous job, taking care of children, and maintaining a household. Others have little physical stress but are under a lot of emotional stress caused both by the way that they perceive events and thoughts they have throughout their days.

How Does Chronic Stress Impact Health?

Anyone who has experienced a period of extreme chronic stress is familiar with the exceptionally negative toll it can take on the body. When we can't recover effectively from the stress response, we break down and become even more intolerant to it. The heightened physical and mental capability

that is produced during the alarm stage comes at a cost—when that cortisol and adrenaline hit the system, your body prioritizes the function of the brain and muscles over digestion, reproduction, and immunity. This can be very helpful when running from a bear, but if it continues to occur chronically, then you end up with imbalances that affect other systems of your body. Some of the researched health consequences of chronic stress are as follows:

- Anxiety
- Cognitive impairment
- Depression
- Digestive upset
- Heart problems
- Sleep problems
- Weight fluctuations

With stress, we have to pay attention to the trickle before it becomes a flood. It starts with things like bills, overscheduling, and not enough time off, and, if left ignored, can result in seemingly unrelated chronic health issues. These consequences are familiar and serve to remind us that unmanaged stress is significant.

What Are Some Causes of Stress?

The causes of stress range from some obvious examples (like an unexpected life event, illness, or change in marital status) to those that are more subtle, like diet, chronic illness, lack of self-care, and fears. We've included a list below to help you pinpoint some of the causes of stress in your life, and help you recognize events that may be contributing to your overall stress burden without your even knowing it (such as having a child go off to college, embarking on a new diet, or remodeling your house).

- **UNEXPECTED MAJOR LIFE EVENT**—This could be a death in the family, an accident, or an acute injury or illness that needs to be handled without warning.

- **DIET**—There are many ways in which diet can be an underlying stressor for your body:
  - Excess sugar
  - Toxins
  - Caffeine
  - Alcohol
  - Food allergy/sensitivity
  - Nutrient deficiency

- **CHRONIC HEALTH PROBLEMS**—those that are not easily resolved with medication or surgery and persist on an ongoing basis:
  - Chronic disease
  - Chronic infection

- **EXPOSURE TO ENVIRONMENTAL TOXINS**—This can be from work, home, water contamination, or personal-care products.

- **EXERCISE**—Both too much or too little exercise can be an underlying source of stress.

- **ALLERGIES**—Environmental allergies chronically impact the immune system as well as interfere with daily life.

- **LACK OF STRESS MANAGEMENT**—not having the means or prioritizing steps to manage stress:
  - Lack of sleep
  - Lack of time off
  - Lack of self-care

- **FAMILY STRESS**—any type of stress related to your immediate and extended family and close friendships:
  - Marital or relational stress
  - Marriage or divorce
  - Addition to the family
  - Family changes
  - In-law troubles

- **FINANCIAL ISSUES**—any type of stress related to your finances:
  - Debt
  - Defaulting on a loan or bankruptcy
  - Lack of resources

- **LEGAL PROBLEMS**—anything from receiving a traffic ticket to being involved in a lawsuit to being incarcerated.

- **EMOTIONAL DIFFICULTIES**—How you react to situations in your daily life can be an underlying cause of stress.

- **MAJOR HABIT CHANGES**—any major changes to your habits, like quitting smoking or trying a new diet.

- **PRESCRIPTION OR OTC MEDICATIONS**—Side effects can cause you significant stress.

- **EMPLOYMENT**—changes to employment status:
  - New employment
  - Ending employment
  - Promotion or demotion
  - Boss/coworker troubles
  - Change in working hours

- **EDUCATION**—changes to schooling or education you may be receiving:

- Starting formal education
- Ending formal education
- Changing institutions

- **CHANGES IN LIVING SITUATION**—changes to your housing or environment:
  - Moving
  - Remodeling
  - Lack of stable living situation

- **FEAR**—Any apprehension or worry that interferes with daily life is a chronic stressor.

- **ATTITUDES AND BELIEFS**—The way you view the world can be a source of stress for your body.

It is important to note again that it isn't just the event or process that is stressful, but it is the way we react to it. While we are in control of *some* of these stressors (like the way we take care of ourselves, our attitudes and beliefs, or the diet we choose to eat), there are others that we have no control over. The point here is not to eliminate every stressor we have in our lives but to control your reaction to the stressors that you don't have control over. Stress will always be a part of our everyday lives. We learn to live healthier and with more resilience by making adjustments where we can.

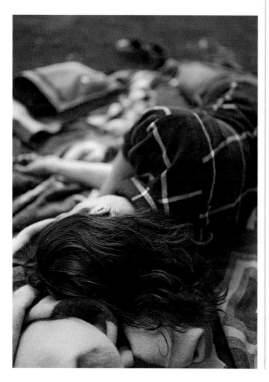

Warning Signs of Burnout and Excessive Stress

Your body has many ways of warning you that the level of stress it is under is not sustainable. Being under a constant barrage of stressful situations without allowing time for restoration and recovery makes it possible to reach a state of chronic burnout and further health disturbances. If you are experiencing any of the symptoms on this list on a regular basis, you should investigate whether your current stress-management routine is adequate for your needs, or if there are any stressors you could potentially eliminate from your life.

- **DIFFICULTY WAKING UP IN THE MORNING**—Cortisol, that hormone secreted by the adrenal glands that is necessary for stimulating your energy levels in the morning, can be lacking due to excessive long-term stress and burnout.

- **FATIGUE DESPITE ADEQUATE SLEEP**—When your need for rest and recovery is greater

(continued on page 120)

WHERE ARE YOU ON THE STRESS-MANAGEMENT SPECTRUM?

This test will help you determine how high a priority stress management is to your healing journey. Give yourself one point for every item that applies to you on the list, and then total your score and see your results at the bottom.

____ I have been experiencing a period of long-term stress.

____ I regularly drive myself to exhaustion.

____ I do not prioritize rest and relaxation.

____ I am easily fatigued.

____ I have a hard time waking up in the morning.

____ I experience energy lows in the afternoon.

____ I tend to gain weight around my middle (hips and thighs).

____ I have one or more chronic illnesses or diseases.

____ I feel that my tolerance to stress is not what it used to be.

____ I suffer from brain fog.

____ My productivity has decreased.

____ I get light-headed when standing up suddenly.

____ I am tired even though I get an adequate amount of sleep.

____ I become light-headed, shaky, or get a headache if I go too long without eating.

____ I have fatigue that is relieved by eating.

____ I rely on caffeine and/or sweets to get through my day.

____ I have a diminished tolerance for people who irritate or bother me.

____ I suffer from intense fears or anxieties.

____ I have feelings of hopelessness.

____ I suffer from frequent colds or flus.

____ It takes me longer than my peers/ family members to recover from a cold or flu.

____ I suffer from panic attacks or nervous breakdowns.

____ I have irregular periods and/or PMS.

____ I crave sweet and/or salty foods.

____ I have a job that causes me a lot of stress.

____ My job requires me to work long hours with little time off.

____ I often worry about work during nonwork hours.

____ I have trouble in my primary relationships.

____ I do not exercise regularly.

____ I don't get enough sleep every night.

____ I don't have any hobbies or activities that I do in my free time.

____ I don't allow myself unstructured time.

____ I don't have a strong social network.

____ I don't practice stress-management or relaxation techniques on a regular basis.

____ I don't have enough income to meet my needs.

1–10 LOW PRIORITY—Good job! It looks like you are already prioritizing your stress management and/or have made a point to remove unneeded stressors in your life.

11–19 MODERATE PRIORITY—Looks like this could use some work! Time to dig in and use the resources that follow in this chapter to start getting your stress under control before it gets worse.

20–35 HIGH PRIORITY—Uh-oh! It appears that your stress level is excessive. Learning how to effectively manage your stress is likely to have a profound impact on your healing journey.

than what your body is getting, you end up feeling tired and unrefreshed.

- **SALTY FOOD CRAVINGS**—Chronic stress can lead to electrolyte imbalances, which cause some people to crave salt.

- **DECREASED ABILITY TO HANDLE STRESSFUL SITUATIONS**—If you have been experiencing prolonged stress, your tolerance for and resilience in subsequent stressful situations decrease considerably.

- **IRREGULAR MENSTRUAL CYCLES AND INCREASED PMS**—Since the body prioritizes stress hormones over sex hormones (and often they are made from the same raw materials), chronic stress leads to imbalances in hormones that can result in irregular cycles, PMS, and even contribute to infertility.

- **FREQUENT COLDS AND FLUS WITH AN INCREASED RECOVERY TIME**—Similar to hormonal balance, the body prioritizes stress hormones over immune function, making it extra hard to fight common colds and other illnesses.

- **LIGHT-HEADEDNESS WHEN STANDING UP**—The electrolyte imbalances that are common with chronic stress often cause you to feel light-headed or dizzy when standing up suddenly.

- **BRAIN FOG**—Excessive stress can cause you to feel like your thinking is consistently foggy and memory can falter.

- **RELIANCE ON CAFFEINE OR SUGAR TO GET THROUGH THE DAY**—Caffeine and sugar both give you a boost when energy levels dip and not being able to go without them can be a sign that your natural energy reserves and resilience to handle stress are lacking.

- **BLOOD-SUGAR SWINGS**—Chronic stress can wreak havoc on your blood-sugar balance, causing you to have energy highs and lows throughout the day.

What Can You Do to Manage Your Stress?

Now that you know all about what stress is and where you are right now in terms of coping with it, we need to start talking about what you can do to manage it. All that previous information won't be useful if it doesn't lead to action. The following list gives you specific ideas to manage stress effectively, with detailed tips and exercises (found on subsequent pages) to accompany some of the ideas.

- **IDENTIFY.** Many of us simply go from 1 day to the next knowing we are stressed out, but not really ever taking time to specifically *identify* what the sources of stress are for us personally. You may have recognized some of your stressors in the examples listed in the preceding section What Are Some Causes of Stress? Take time to sit down and write the most complete list you can of everything that you perceive as stress in your life. Your list should include obvious things like a job loss and less clear things that are a source of strain, like that stack of paperwork on the kitchen table.

- **EXAMINE.** Honestly *examine* your daily routine. Ask yourself if you are doing all you can in terms of lifestyle habits that

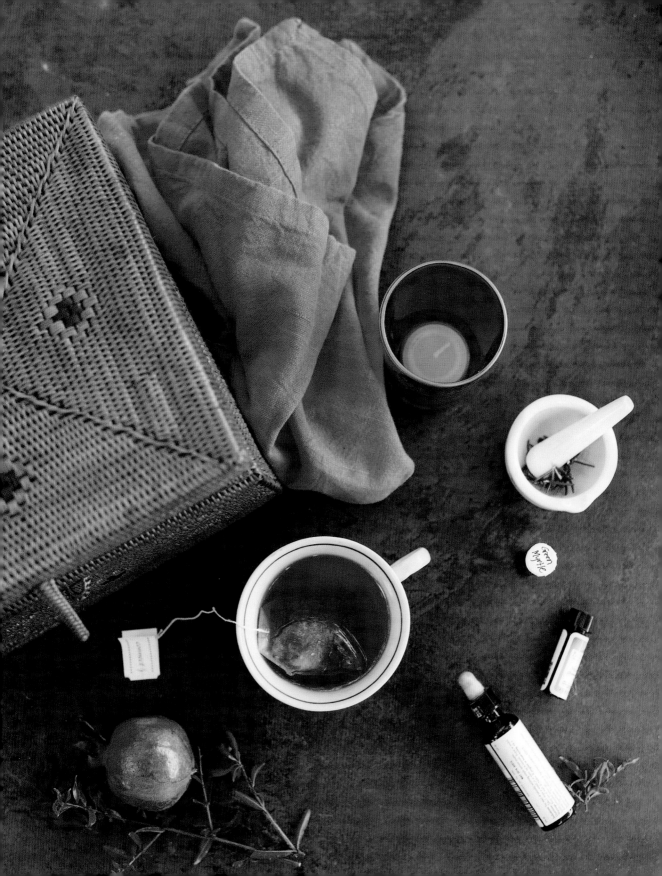

greatly influence your stress load. Eating well, getting enough sleep, and exercising regularly have an enormous impact on your ability to cope with stress, and having exceptionally poor habits in any of these areas can be a stressor in itself. Be sure to check in with yourself to see if measures to improve these basic areas could make a difference.

- **ELIMINATE.** Evaluate sources of stress that can simply be removed from your life. We are not able to control everything we may face, but there are some things that are within our control. Where it is possible for you, *eliminate* sources of stress without guilt or shame. This might mean, for instance, saying no to interactions with "energy robbers." "Energy robbers" is the name coined by James L. Wilson, ND, DC, PhD, author of *Adrenal Fatigue*, to describe people, conditions, and even foods that drain us. Another example might be that you stop connecting on a particular social media platform. An honest look at what can be completely taken off your plate is a huge stride forward in managing your stress. *(See the Tips for Maintaining a Healthy Relationship with Technology section, page 126).*

- **PRIORITIZE.** An immense stressor for many of us is being overwhelmed. With so many items on the daily to-do list, it is inevitable that we find ourselves paralyzed on where to direct our attention. It can be helpful to assess where these items fall in terms of importance and proactively *prioritize* in order to accomplish them. The mantra here is, "Manage your to-do list, don't let it manage you."

- **PRACTICE.** It is great to find ways of eliminating stress, but we must also add healthy stress-reducing activities into our lives. Carving out time to pursue fun and relaxing activities that help counterbalance the stress that cannot be eliminated is vital. On the following page is a list of possible habits for you to *practice* using on a daily, weekly/monthly, or seasonally/yearly basis. You will find that some of them are easy and straightforward, while others will take conscious effort on your part to schedule or develop, for instance practicing mindfulness. (See "Habits to Cultivate" on page 124 and the Mindfulness Tips section on page 127.)

- **REFRAME.** Some stressors, despite how large they may be, can be greatly diminished when we *reframe* our internal thoughts around them. Analyzing how we think, feel, and talk to ourselves about a source of stress can be a powerful tool, especially if we take it a step further and challenge those thoughts with a new dialogue. For example, the author Malcolm Gladwell, in his book *David and Goliath,* encourages readers to recognize some obstacles in life as "desirable difficulties," a term used to describe unfavorable situations that result in advantages for the person facing them. Learning to see things in a different light can be a profound stress-management

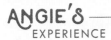

Actively managing my stress is an ongoing process for me. Just when I think I have it all mastered, something new comes up, and finding the best way to tackle it so that stress doesn't derail my health becomes my priority once again. Of all the ideas on how to manage stress, how to "reframe" was the breakthrough for me. Analyzing how I thought, felt, and spoke to myself about certain sources of stress was huge in reducing my reactions. When I took it further and began using new words to describe challenges in my life, it transformed me. Realizing I had the power to structure my thought processes for increased positivity was amazing!

tool. See resilienceacademy.com for practical guidance on how to reframe.

- **ACCEPT.** There are occasions when the most positive step you can take in addressing a source of stress is learning to *accept* it. This can be a very uncomfortable process, but sometimes plainly acknowledging the reality of a stressor that you cannot change, like a troublesome family situation or illness, and letting go is the only way forward. In these cases, it can be meaningful to regularly check in with yourself about what valuable lessons you may be gaining by learning to live with the stressor.

- **ALTER.** The most radical idea is saved for last. You may find that some stress cannot be managed with any of the other ideas presented here and that continuing to tolerate it is also not an option. If that is the case, it is time to *alter* your situation, even if the change itself will present stress. Perhaps your job has become absolutely unbearable or you are very unhappy where you live.

Maybe a relationship has grown toxic. With these kinds of stressors, considering a major lifestyle change is in order. Start to carefully plan how to make necessary adjustments in the least-disruptive and most timely way possible, while leaning on your support network through the change.

THE IMPORTANCE OF SELF-CARE

Self-care is the choice to prioritize activities that are essential to protecting your well-being. While we would all agree that self-preservation is a natural and appropriate instinct, the truth is that the more proactive version of preservation, self-care, is kind of a sensitive topic, especially in the United States. We tend to have a nearly overpowering work ethic, at the expense of equal time given to caring for ourselves. Even though there are a great many resources and much talk about how important it is to practice good self-care, the underlying message in our society is often "self-care is selfish."

The truth is best stated by author and educator Parker J. Palmer, PhD, "Self-care is never a selfish act—it is simply good stewardship of the only gift I have, the gift I was put on Earth to offer others. Anytime we can listen to true self and give the care it requires, we do it not only for ourselves, but for the many others whose lives we touch." We sometimes describe this topic as the "plane crash scenario." If your plane is going down and oxygen masks are required, you must first put on your own mask before you can help the person sitting next to you. Some people might say, "But what if that person sitting next to me is my partner or child?" It doesn't matter how much more important the person next to

you seems to be, without your own oxygen flowing, you will quickly lose consciousness and be completely unable to help yourself or anyone else. It may be the case in life that the "person sitting next to you" is someone totally dependent on you, like a child or elderly parent, which makes "putting on your oxygen" even more crucial. You will not be able to uphold your responsibility to care for anyone else if you have not first upheld your responsibility to care for yourself.

Don't undervalue self-care or allow guilt to creep in when you prioritize it. Eating well, sleeping deeply, managing stress, and other practices that provide a well-rounded holistic self-care routine are

HABITS TO CULTIVATE

DAILY HABITS

- Mindfulness or spiritual practice
  - Prayer
  - Breathwork
  - Meditation
- Creative activities
  - Art
  - Playing music
  - Creative writing
- Light exercise
  - Walking
  - Yoga
- Unstructured time
- Self-care
  - Bathing
  - Diffusing essential oils
- Reading

- Listening to music
- Playing a game
- Delegating tasks
- Journaling

WEEKLY/MONTHLY HABITS

- Two work-free days a week
- Acupuncture
- Massage
- Talk therapy
- Gathering with your community
- Caretaking

SEASONALLY/YEARLY OR AS NEEDED

- Vacation
- Time off from work
- Sabbatical

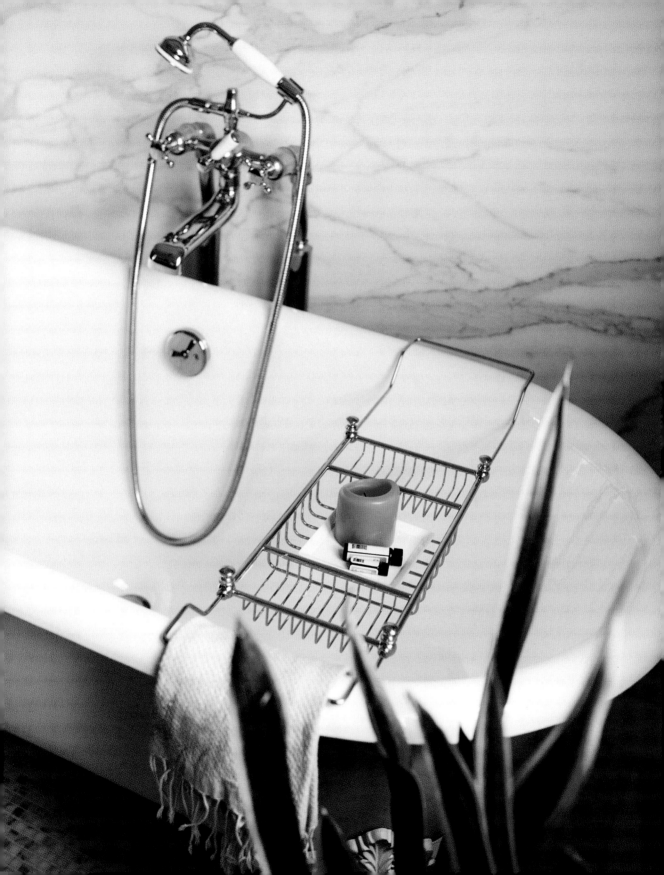

smart investments in not only you but all those who depend on you. This is especially true if you have an autoimmune disease, since anything you can do to support good health minimizes the impact of the chronic nature of your illness. It's just plain smart to dedicate time and resources to the "maintenance" of you!

Tips for Maintaining a Healthy Relationship with Technology

The modern technology that we have access to is nothing short of revolutionary, and can be both an incredible tool as well as a chronic stressor for our bodies. It isn't the particular technology itself that is "good" or "bad," but the habits that we develop around how we use it. If you are someone who sleeps with your phone interrupting you with a series of notifications throughout the night, checks email first thing when you wake up or before bed, and cannot go to a social event without pulling out your phone every 5 minutes, you may have some work to do in cultivating a healthier relationship with technology.

As we described in Chapter 4, screens found on televisions, computers, and devices such as tablets and smartphones all emit blue-spectrum light that is disruptive to your circadian rhythm. Exposure to this spectrum of light after dark can be a stressor for your body, as it disrupts your natural hormonal balance and interferes with sleep. This isn't the only way technology is a stressor—being connected to your work and social life 24/7 can be incredibly depleting. Our brains need time off from the constant barrage of to-do lists, emails, messages, updates, and notifications.

Sometimes, it feels like drinking from a fire hose! If you are looking for some tips to help cultivate a more *useful* and less *stressful* relationship with technology, follow these guidelines.

- Limit your social media use to communicating and sharing; don't use it as a "time-filler" or as a replacement for activity when bored.
- Avoid screens an hour or two before bed.
- Charge your devices outside your bedroom.
- Minimize the use of notifications on device applications (email, social media, etc.).
- Check emails only a few times a day and don't leave email applications open while working.
- Avoid checking email right before bed or right upon waking.
- Avoid replacing one-on-one time or phone calls with social media contact.
- Avoid watching TV or using a device while eating meals or having a conversation.
- Take a "technology detox" or a "social media vacation" periodically.
- Avoid spending so much time with technology that you don't have any time for real-life activity.

The Autoimmune Wellness Handbook

- Leave your devices at home or turned off in your pocket to have a richer, more mindful experience without the distraction.

Mindfulness Tips

Mindfulness is all about recognizing the little things, something that is all too often absent from our busy, overscheduled modern lives. It is important to find ways to actively check in with yourself and ask questions about the moment you are experiencing. This can help you connect more often and more deeply to your life, as well as help you shape and direct your thoughts, rather than allow them to overwhelm you and contribute to stress. Use the list of questions below to help you brainstorm some ways in which you can practice greater awareness of your present experience.

- While I'm washing dishes, what does the temperature of the water feel like?
- While I'm talking with a loved one, am I noticing the special qualities of his/her voice?
- While I'm out for a daily walk, what small details of the scenery have changed today?
- While I'm eating my meal, what textures and aromas do I find satisfying?
- While I'm sitting down at my desk, what is energizing me about the work ahead?
- While I'm driving, what am I noticing about the road conditions?
- While I'm lying down for the night, how does my body feel?

MICKEY'S EXPERIENCE

Of all of the areas of stress management, cultivating a healthy relationship with technology is one that I continue to struggle with, even today. I am constantly feeling the need to check email, Facebook, and other notifications, waiting for tasks to "drip" in, and cluttering my brain up with future to-dos. When I am not managing well in this area, I find myself feeling frazzled, stressed, not sleeping well, and more likely to make poor lifestyle or dietary choices. Little habits like only checking email twice a day during work hours, only checking social media once a day at predetermined times, and never checking email or social media first thing in the morning or before bed go a long way at helping me stay balanced. I also find that my connections with my spouse and family are much more meaningful when I am not distracted by this technology. It is a continual struggle, but I find when I give attention to these practices, my health flourishes.

- While I'm playing with my child, am I noticing the special aspects of his/her face?
- While I'm listening to music, am I noticing a certain instrument or voice?
- While I'm cooking dinner, what can I imagine about the farmers who grew my food?

Don't Let Stress Management Stress You Out!

It seems like a lot, right? Managing your stress is a big job, it's true. It takes vigilance

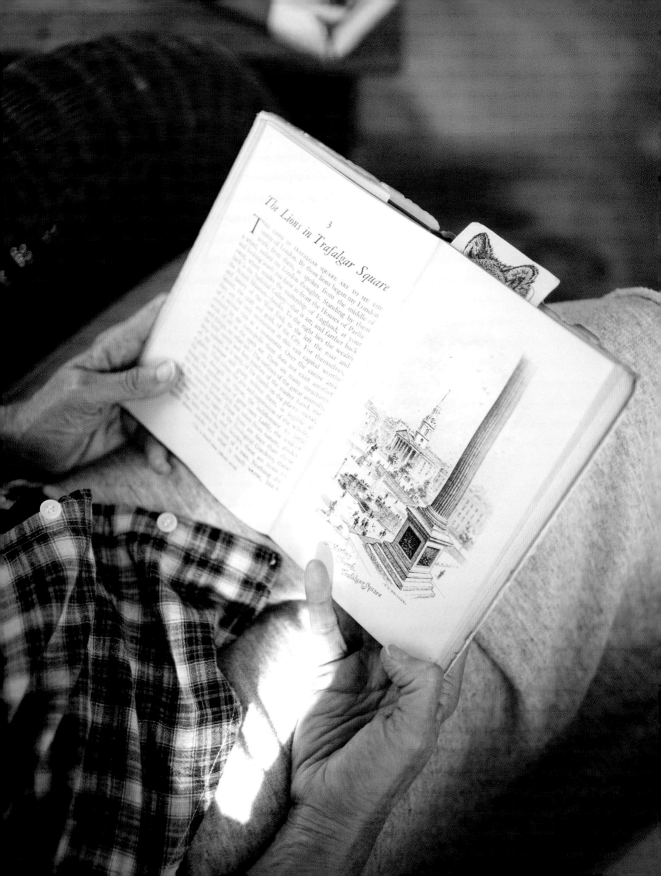

and commitment and time. Certain techniques for managing stress might not feel like good matches for you. Do you find yourself dreading your date with that next guided meditation module you've been working on? It shouldn't be that way!

Try your best to take things a step at a time, slowly changing your mind-set around stress management and then putting new tools into use. Consider planning "taste tests," where you choose two or three different techniques and then try them short-term (no pressure to commit!) just to see if they feel comfortable and enjoyable to you. Just because half the world is going nuts for yoga doesn't mean that it has to work for you, too. Maybe a few hours a week in a workshop building model airplanes is more your style. Chapter 9 offers ideas for how to incorporate stress management slowly, making the habit of using these techniques more manageable. Bottom line here—don't let stress management stress you out! That's totally not the zen thing to do!

CALL TO ACTION

The purpose of this chapter is to show you that, after nourishment and rest, learning to *breathe* is crucially important to a life.

Perfecting your approach to stress reduction is no small task. It's also not a task we ever finish. Managing your stress is like doing the laundry or taking out the trash: It must be repeated regularly or it will pile up and have negative consequences on you and your health. Mountains of laundry are unsightly and mounds of trash are smelly! Unmanaged stress leaves people and their bodies in a very similar disarray.

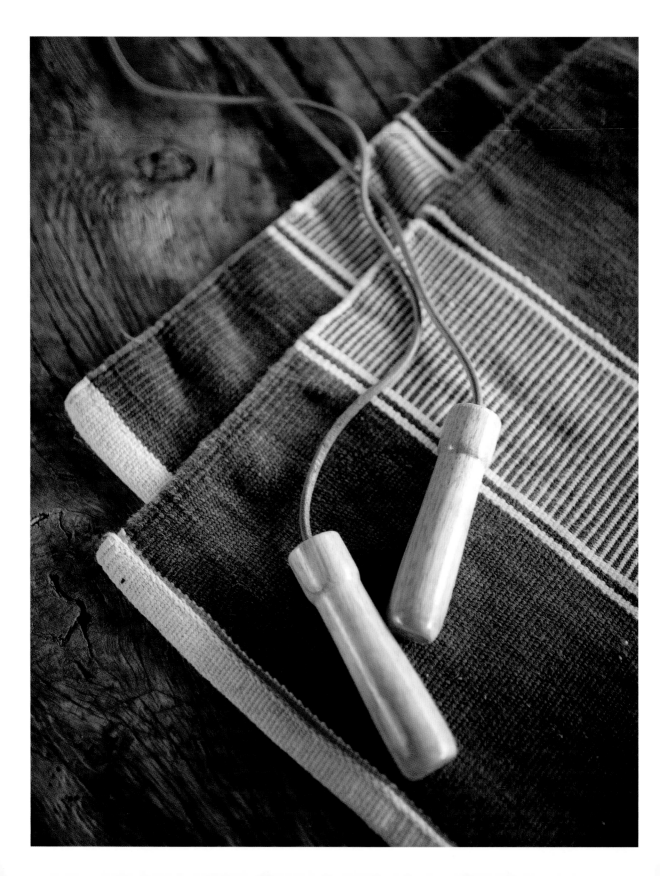

CHAPTER 6

Move

"Lack of activity destroys the good condition of every human being, while movement and methodical physical exercise save it and preserve it."—PLATO

OUR ANCESTORS SPENT MOST OF THEIR time on their feet, going about the daily tasks that afforded them food and shelter. While civilization has brought about radical changes that have positively impacted the way we live, the extent to which it has enabled us to be physically inactive is causing disastrous consequences in our health. The human body is designed to move! Unless you are a farmer, you don't have to worry about tending your crops or feeding your livestock. Today, you can get your groceries delivered to your door without even leaving the comfort of your couch. This may seem like a convenient solution, but the way modern society outsources many of the physical tasks necessary for life takes a toll.

The minimum amount of weekly exercise recommended by the Centers for Disease Control and Prevention (CDC) for healthy adults is 2½ hours of moderate exercise (like walking) and 2 sessions of full-body strengthening exercises, or 1¼ hours of intense exercise (like running) and 2 sessions of full-body strengthening exercises. Only 1 in 5 Americans currently meets these recommendations, meaning that 80 percent of us are not getting the *minimum* amount of movement we need to be healthy. In addition, many experts argue that the CDC's recommendations are only scratching the surface of what your body's true movement needs are.

If you have an autoimmune disease, getting the movement you need is likely to be more difficult. It's a shame, when studies show that those suffering from autoimmune diseases who get regular exercise have a higher quality of life and mental health than those who don't, even when physical limitations like pain or fatigue are accounted for. Even though it can be difficult getting past these barriers, managing to be active enough provides us with the enhanced health and well-being that is necessary for living with chronic illness. In this chapter, you'll learn why you need to prioritize movement as well as find some creative solutions for getting started and integrating activity into your routine.

WHY DO YOU NEED TO MOVE?

The primary motivator for most people to exercise is the positive physical changes that come with being fit—weight loss, muscle gain, and an improved body composition. Most often, we are motivated by a desire to be thin and look attractive, neither of which is a clear indicator of true health. There are other, and we'd argue, more compelling reasons for making sure you are moving your body in a way that is supportive of vibrant health, and not in the pursuit of an unrealistic body image. Here are some of the biggest reasons why you need to make movement a priority.

- **IT PREVENTS DISEASE.** Those who exercise regularly have a lower chance of developing heart disease and diabetes, having a stroke, getting certain kinds of cancers, becoming obese, and developing other health problems.

- **IT STRENGTHENS BONES.** Certain types of movement (like walking and running) increase bone mineral density and promote bone strength, preventing osteoporosis (bone loss).

- **IT STRENGTHENS YOUR BODY.** Regular exercise strengthens your muscles, tendons, ligaments, and joints, making everyday activities easier to achieve.

- **IT MAINTAINS A STRONG AND HEALTHY HEART.** Regular exercise increases aerobic capacity (the ability to take in and use oxygen) and lowers risk factors leading to heart problems.

- **IT PROMOTES THE FLOW OF LYMPH.** Your lymphatic system, a network of vessels and nodes that have immune functions, lacks a pump (like the heart for the cardiovascular system) and is dependent on the movement of your muscles and joints to move fluids around the body. This is necessary for proper detoxification and immune function.

- **IT PROMOTES FLEXIBILITY.** Especially when you engage in a wide variety of movements, exercise promotes a healthy range of motion in your joints and flexibility in your muscles.

- **IT HELPS MANAGE STRESS.** Moving appropriately can be a great outlet for stress management, not to mention a whole lot of fun!

- **IT IMPROVES SLEEP.** Physical activity can increase sleep quality and duration.

- **IT INCREASES CONCENTRATION AND FOCUS.** Those who exercise tend to be more productive and on-task than those who don't.

- **IT KEEPS YOU HAPPY.** Exercise promotes emotional well-being, happiness, and reduces anxiety and depression.

As you can see, engaging in an exercise routine can help with a couple of the factors we've already talked about in Chapters 4 and 5—Rest and Breathe. This should be motivation to take small steps to make

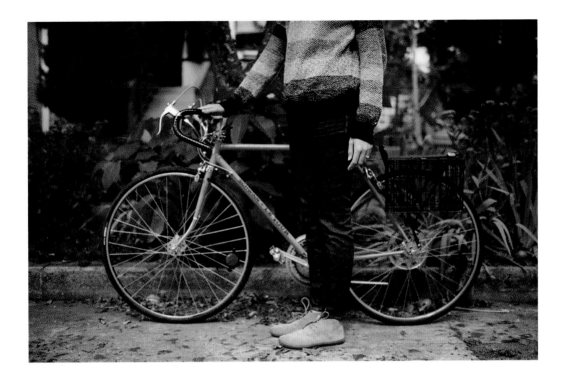

improvements in all of these areas instead of just one, as they are likely to have a positive impact on each other and result in a more profound shift (for putting it all together, see Chapter 9).

WHY IS EXERCISE DIFFICULT FOR THOSE WITH AUTOIMMUNE DISEASE?

Those with autoimmune disease tend to be more inactive than healthy individuals, for a variety of reasons. You may suffer from barriers to movement stemming from the symptoms of your disease, like joint pain, muscle pain, and fatigue. Or, you could suffer from mental health issues, like depression, which can function as a barrier to movement because of the lack of motivation

that comes with it. Your key player may not have informed you on ways you can safely incorporate movement into your routine or may have just ignored the topic altogether. Family and friends may make the assumption that you can't or don't want to engage in physical activity because they have a limited understanding of your disease. All of these factors can add up, making it even more difficult for you to find an exercise routine that you love and is supportive of your healing process.

Even though those of us with autoimmune disease may face unique challenges when considering adding movement into our routines, it is worthwhile not to ignore this aspect of the healing journey. At the very minimum, movement is necessary for essential body processes, as outlined on page 132. If you are in the beginning stages of an autoimmune disease, incorporating exercise may help slow the progression of your disease and keep you healthier long-term. A 2015 literature review found that the most common barriers to exercise for those with rheumatoid arthritis were the very issues that research shows are *positively* impacted by exercise—pain and fatigue! Often, the very reasons we aren't able to exercise can be improved by exercise itself.

Before you lace up those running shoes and head out the door, we'd like to get the message across that exercise, or *movement* as we like to call it, for those with autoimmune disease may look different than what you typically think of. While intense activities like working out at the gym, running, and cycling are all great forms of exercise, you may not be capable of those kinds of workouts. And that is okay! We'll be offering some creative, autoimmune-friendly solutions to the movement problem as we work through this.

MOVING TOO MUCH?

While it may seem that, by and large, our society has a problem with people moving too little, the truth is that there is a sizable problem with people moving too much. You may think there's no downside to moving, that there is no "too much," but there are repercussions. As Sarah Ballantyne, PhD, points out in her book *The Paleo Approach*, the benefits of exercise can be measured in a U-shape. Excessive movement leads to disregulated cortisol (the stress hormone from Chapter 4), increased susceptibility to immune-related diseases, and leaky gut. Overexercise for a person with autoimmune disease can be harmful because of inflammation and immune suppression, which increase symptoms of disease.

Signs of overdoing it, beyond the obvious like fatigue, pain, decreased performance, and the need for increased recovery time, can range from insomnia to low libido to loss of menstruation and even depression. You might also notice that you are more susceptible to illness, especially upper-respiratory infections. Those with autoimmune disease might experience more frequent flares. So why do people feel compelled to move excessively? The reasons are varied and in many cases, overlapping.

- **WEIGHT-LOSS STRUGGLES.** Some people overdo it in an attempt to shed real or imagined extra pounds, believing that if they can just work out enough, they'll reach the "perfect" weight. In some cases, being overweight might actually be related to an underlying health problem that must first be addressed and can't be exercised away. For instance, weight gain is often a symptom of Hashimoto's thyroiditis.

- **BODY-IMAGE STRUGGLES.** Struggling with body image very often overlaps weight-loss struggles. Simply put, a person may believe that her body is not acceptable as it is and feel a need to "sculpt" it into a "perfect" shape.

The Autoimmune Wellness Handbook

- **CARDIO OBSESSION.** This particular form of overdoing it, using long-duration aerobic exercise or cardio, can also go hand in hand with the weight-loss struggle. A person may believe that the fastest way to weight loss is to burn as many calories as possible, sometimes running, hitting the treadmill or elliptical machine, or attending grueling stationary cycling classes, to the point of exhaustion.

- **FAD WORKOUTS.** Occasionally, people feel pressure to join the latest workout craze, even if the particular routine is too much for them or just not a good fit. It might be that the need to keep up with friends who are into P90X, CrossFit, or Bikram yoga is driving a person beyond what is beneficial for him.

- **STRESS MANAGEMENT.** In some cases, a person may not feel that he has any other effective methods of managing his stress. He may rely solely and excessively on exercising as his outlet, rather than looking for ways to reduce stress or manage it with a balance of active and resting methods.

- **ACHIEVEMENT FOCUS.** Athletes can be particularly vulnerable to doing excessive exercise that is focused on achievement. If they see their only value in an external reward, like running the most marathons or winning the most weight-lifting competitions, the tendency can be to overtrain.

- **EXERCISE ADDICTION.** Exercise addiction, also called "activity disorder," is real. This is excessive, purposeless physical activity that goes beyond usual routines and

MICKEY'S EXPERIENCE

I am a recovering activity addict. My response to the early signs of autoimmune disease like fatigue, joint pain, and lack of recovery was actually to push my body and increase my workouts in an attempt to manage symptoms and stress. Back then, I didn't own a car and cycled to work, lifted weights a few days at the gym, attended a few yoga classes, a spin class or two, and ran nearly every day. I would go through phases of intense exercise and then burn out, crashing for a few days or weeks, and then start the cycle all over again. A huge wake-up call for me was when I could no longer ride my bike up a large hill on my daily commute. I could not believe that with all of the exercise and strength-training that I would actually be getting weaker. What I was experiencing was the early warning signs of muscle wasting and fatigue.

Recovery for me meant reevaluating all of these habits and replacing them with more sustainable, health-supporting activities. That being said, I still constantly have to catch myself from falling into the old habit of moving too much. Instead of managing my stress through intense workouts, I choose qigong, yoga, and walking. I no longer aspire to run marathons or do century bike rides. Instead, I have made a commitment to move my body in a way that strengthens it but does not cause excess harm or stress.

impairs rather than improves health and well-being. A person facing exercise addiction is uncomfortable with rest and will work out to the exclusion of almost all other areas of her life, even to the point of danger.

Tips for Those Who Move Too Much

If you find yourself tending toward moving too much, these are some tips that will help you tone it down a notch and enable your body to heal.

- **LOOK FOR ROOT CAUSES OF WEIGHT-LOSS RESISTANCE.** If you have trouble losing weight and use intense exercise to manage it, you may want to talk to your key player about underlying health issues that could be standing in the way. For instance, the lack of thyroid hormone in Hashimoto's thyroiditis can lead to weight-loss resistance that is difficult or impossible to "out-exercise."

- **FIND BODY ACCEPTANCE.** Your body is perfect just the way it is. Movement should be done for optimal health, not to force our bodies into an unrealistic mold.

- **FIND A GENTLER OR MORE APPROPRIATE WAY TO WORK OUT.** Swap out some of those high-intensity workouts for activities that are easier on your body. For instance, you can trade your 30-minute run for an hour walk, or your CrossFit workout for power yoga.

- **GIVE YOUR BODY MORE TIME TO RECOVER.** Especially if you find yourself feeling sore and fatigued on a regular basis, give yourself a day or two between more intense activities.

- **LOOK FOR A MORE APPROPRIATE WAY TO MANAGE STRESS.** If you are looking to intense exercise to help manage your stress, try finding a stress-management activity that is also restorative. Turn down the volume on your routine and go for a walk, do some stretching, or dance. There are ways you can manage your stress through movement without overdoing it.

- **LET GO OF ACHIEVEMENT.** Prioritize the goal to best support your body's health instead of running that marathon or competing in a bike race. Letting go of the idea that you always need to be achieving an external reward will give you more space to just be who you are and move in a way that feels right.

- **GET HELP FOR EXERCISE ADDICTION OR OBSESSIVE TENDENCIES.** If you find yourself addicted to or obsessed with exercise, you should be evaluated by a professional and have her help guide your recovery. Common in those who have struggled with eating disorders in the past, this is a sign that you may need some additional support to break the addictive cycle.

Fitspo and Shame

Fitspiration or "Fitspo" is a buzzword that stands for "fitness inspiration." It is the sharing of images on social media of active, strong, usually lean women (and occasionally men), along with an inspiring message promoting exercise and/or diet in order to achieve an "ideal" body. The messages say things like "Strong is the new skinny" or "Puking is acceptable, quitting is not." Others have slogans across a sexy female body that read "Don't quit until you're proud."

Fitness inspiration is supposed to motivate people toward health, but the images accompanying the messages are often extremely unrealistic. The messages themselves often border on bullying, like, "What's your excuse?" or "Your body can handle the pain, tell your mind to shut up." The idea that we cannot be good enough unless we have achieved the unattainable or worked ourselves to the point of burnout is enormously harmful.

The insinuation with Fitspo is that you should feel a great deal of shame if you don't measure up to the standard being presented. This can be particularly damaging to those with autoimmune disease, who may already be dealing with negative messaging from those around them about whether or not they are "really sick." Working toward increased health is a worthy goal, but it need not carry with it such a destructive burden. Be alert to this cultural misinformation about fitness, and challenge those negative thoughts with balance. Find the right level of movement for your body, autoimmune disease appropriately accounted for, and enjoy being active. No exposure to abusive "motivation" required!

Moving Too Little?

The benefits of getting enough physical activity are well understood. Our bodies were made to move and move often. That regular movement is key to achieving and maintaining good health. Just like there is a downside to moving too much, the other side of the U-shaped curve reveals the negative impact of too little movement. When you aren't getting enough physical activity, your immune system is compromised, your resistance to stress is decreased, and your circadian rhythm is easily thrown off.

Despite the obvious benefits and clear disadvantages, for some, getting enough exercise into their lives is a serious challenge. These challenges can range from perceived barriers to significant physical impediments. Especially for those of us with autoimmune disease, it can be helpful to explore the reasons that we may be moving too little.

Common Barriers

Most people find that their barriers to movement fall into the "excuses" category. These barriers have simple solutions that can be easily applied.

- Lack of time
- Boredom or dislike of exercise setting
- Loneliness or lack of motivation
- Bad weather
- Working a desk job or long hours
- Not seeing results

Complex Barriers

Sometimes, barriers to movement are not as easily resolved and may involve physical or valid psychological limitations that require more-sensitive solutions. In some of these cases, consulting with a personal trainer who specializes in autoimmune disease, mobility training, and/or body positivity may be helpful.

- **PAIN/INJURY.** This is the first big factor that often comes up for people with autoimmune disease. Moving, especially with diseases like rheumatoid arthritis, might actually hurt . . . *a lot!* Autoimmune diseases that affect mobility might also contribute to being easily or frequently injured.

- **FATIGUE.** This is the second big factor that comes up for those of us with autoimmune disease. You may find that your disease leaves you with only enough energy for very basic activity, and sometimes just showering takes all you have for that day. Sometimes, when you start a routine, you find that you are quickly depleted and unable to finish.

- **WRONG INTENSITY LEVEL.** Due to some of the cultural misinformation, as well as the influence of fad workouts, it can be hard to determine the right intensity level of physical activity for you. This may be particularly true if you are coming from a previously athletic lifestyle or from a completely sedentary lifestyle. In both cases, you may be out of touch with how your body communicates what is appropriate

versus inappropriate. See "Exercise Assessment" on page 143 for help figuring out if a workout is appropriate for you.

- **INTERNAL BELIEFS, FEAR, OR SHAME.** It is not unusual for autoimmune disease to leave us with some strong inner thought processes around movement. You may believe that you are not capable of increasing your fitness level, be afraid of the pain or injury you've associated with moving and your disease in the past, or feel ashamed that you aren't able to be active at a previous level or at the level expected by healthier family members or friends.

- **FEELING OF BEING OVERWHELMED ABOUT WHERE TO START.** What program should you be doing anyway? It can be hard to determine what kind of routine is ideal when you are first beginning to improve your fitness level, particularly if you have a disease to factor into your decision. Feeling overwhelmed can lead to a state of paralysis, where you find it hard to move forward and so remain underactive.

Tips for Those Who Don't Move Enough

If you find yourself tending toward not moving enough, here are some tips to help you troubleshoot the barriers that are keeping you from activity and find some solutions.

- **SWITCH IT UP!** If you find yourself getting bored easily, you don't have to do the same activities day after day. Maybe Monday you go for a long walk, Tuesday you take a yoga

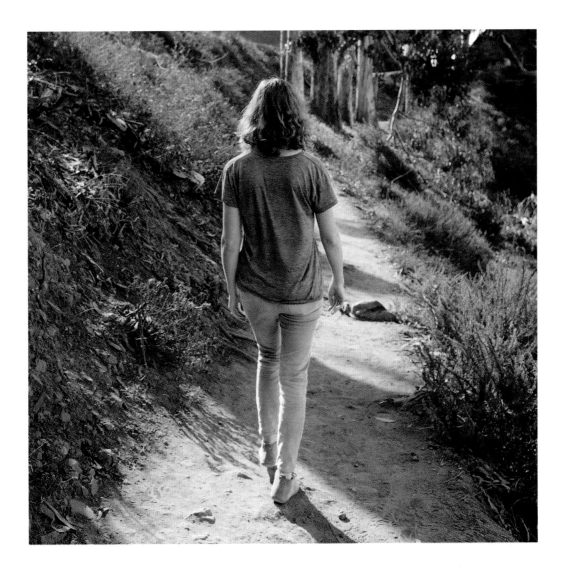

class, and Wednesday you put on some music and dance around the house while you get some chores done.

- **FIND A BUDDY**. You may find that having a partner to exercise with motivates you to continue with your routine, plus you get a boost from the social activity. If your spouse, friend, or neighbor doesn't want to get active

with you, look for a suitable partner via an online network or in your community.

- **HAVE A BACKUP**. If your workout is dependent on the weather, have a backup in mind in case conditions are not favorable. For instance, if you always walk in your neighborhood, have a yoga mat and a DVD at home in case rain interrupts your plans.

- **USE A STANDING OR TREADMILL DESK AND TAKE MOVEMENT BREAKS**. If you sit at a computer all day, why not try a standing, treadmill, or modular (combination) desk to keep your position changing throughout the day?

- **ENROLL IN A CLASS**. For those who have issues with commitment, sometimes enrolling in a series or class will help motivate you to participate and prioritize movement.

- **TAKE ACTION ON PSYCHOLOGICAL AND PHYSICAL BARRIERS**. Your autoimmune disease may cause issues with mobility, and although things may change for the better, sometimes this aspect is out of your control. Working with a practitioner who is experienced with mobility issues caused by autoimmune disease can be helpful in determining the types of movement that are less likely to cause pain or injury. You can also do something about your internal beliefs, fear, shame, and feeling overwhelmed about exercise. Look for affirming or constructive ways to address these issues on your own or with the help of a therapist.

- **AVOID FEELING OVERWHELMED**. Start with one type of activity that sounds enjoyable and is well matched to your fitness level. You can always change if you don't like it or feel like it is not enough/too much for your body at this time.

- **LISTEN TO YOUR BODY**. Working out should make you feel tired and sore to a certain extent, but you need to be constantly checking in with yourself to make sure you aren't doing too much too soon. When in doubt, be extra cautious, start slow, and ramp up the intensity at a comfortable rate.

- **GET HELP FROM AN EXPERT**. If you feel unsure about starting an exercise routine, there is always the option to work one-on-one

ANGIE'S EXPERIENCE

Not moving enough hasn't always been an issue for me. Prior to developing my autoimmune diseases, I enjoyed hiking and even longer backpacking trips. While it was a challenge, the beautiful walks in nature and the pride in carrying everything I needed on my own back were huge rewards, not to mention the chance to connect with friends. As my body became more and more malnourished with undiagnosed celiac disease, I had less and less ability to perform physically at previous levels. I started noticing that I was breathless, light-headed, and shaky only 10 to 15 minutes into a workout of any kind. I even remember my husband urging me to eat energy bars not only following a workout, but even *before* doing anything! I simply had no reserves, and I became afraid of experiencing those sensations. Eventually, I avoided movement almost altogether. To this day, I struggle with movement on the autoimmune wellness journey. Although I am not as debilitated as I once was, I find myself having to work hard to overcome the fears that I felt around exertion while I was sick, and I often find myself trying to tackle a sense of being overwhelmed about restoring physical fitness. The journey is complex, and some areas take us years to master.

WHERE ARE YOU ON THE MOVEMENT SPECTRUM?

This test will help you determine how high of a priority movement is to your healing journey. Give yourself one point for every item on the list that applies, and then total your score and see your results at the bottom.

____ I sit for 7 or more hours per day.

____ I get less than 1 hour total of moderate physical activity per day (like walking).

____ I always drive to work, school, or other commitments.

____ I don't spend any time stretching during the week.

____ I don't do any activities that build muscle, like lifting heavy objects or bodyweight exercises, like pushups or squats.

____ I have a health condition that restricts my ability to move.

____ My work doesn't require me to be on my feet at all during the day.

____ I don't make time to exercise during the week.

____ My free time is centered around sedentary activities (like watching TV).

____ I don't enjoy exercise.

SCORING: Any score higher than 4 means that you may need to prioritize getting more movement throughout your day. To ensure that you aren't overdoing it, see "Exercise Assessment" on page 143.

---

with a personal trainer. Ideally, you would look for someone who has experience working with autoimmune disease, mobility training, and/or a focus on body positivity.

EXERCISE IDEAS FOR THOSE WITH CHRONIC ILLNESS

Although some top-level athletes suffer from autoimmune disease and still find themselves able to perform at a high level (like Venus Williams), this is rare and by far an exception to the rule. If you have an autoimmune disease, chances are that you are going to do better with moderate exercise instead of intense exercise. The good news is that this moderate exercise has been shown to be just as health promoting as intense activity, without the risk of

injury, burnout, and stress. Here are some ideas that can get you started.

● **WALKING**—No movement is as simple and innate as walking, and the possibilities are endless. You can walk anywhere and from a few minutes to a few hours a day, depending on your fitness and strength level. We believe this is the ideal activity for those with autoimmune disease—see The Benefits of Walking section on page 144 for more details.

● **YOGA**—A practice that integrates breathwork and stretching that promotes flexibility and strength, as well as relaxation. There are many different types of yoga, ranging from gentle and restorative to intense and strength-building.

- **PILATES**—A series of core exercises originally developed to be rehabilitative that improve strength and flexibility.

- **QIGONG**—An integrated Chinese system of posture, movement, and meditation that can help with strength, flexibility, and promoting relaxation.

- **TAI CHI**—A Chinese martial arts practice that uses slower movements and helps with balance, focus, and strength.

- **STRETCHING**—Any activity that focuses on lengthening the muscles. Stretching can be done on its own or as a component of another exercise like yoga or Pilates.

- **SWIMMING**—Getting exercise while immersed in water can be less strenuous and easier on the joints. Swimming or water aerobics can range from gentle to intense depending on the type of workout you'd like to receive.

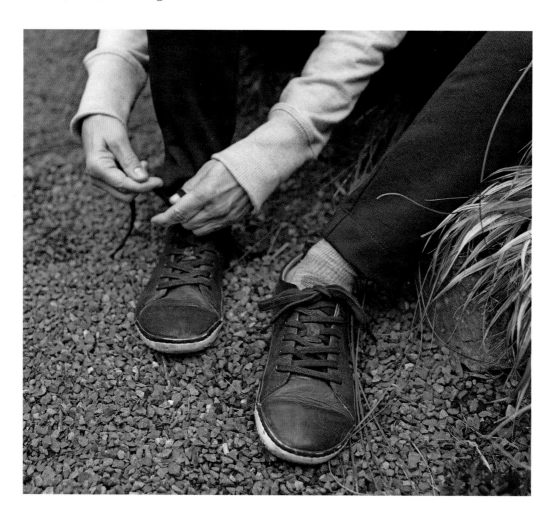

- **HIKING**—Walking on a nature trail or in the outdoors can be an excellent way to get some movement. It can be something as simple as a flat trail around a body of water or as strenuous as backpacking for a couple of days in the wilderness.

- **DANCING**—Put on some of your favorite tunes and move your body! Dancing is one of the most fun and enjoyable ways to get your daily movement.

- **LEISURELY CYCLING**—Take your bike for a spin around the neighborhood or make the commitment to start riding to work.

- **MARTIAL ARTS**—There are many different types of martial arts practices that focus to varying degrees on strength, flexibility, coordination, meditation, and breathwork and can be an enjoyable and challenging way to get movement into your routine.

- **REBOUNDING**—Use a mini rebounding trampoline to gently bounce, getting a maximum workout for minimum effort.

As any stay-at-home-parent can attest, being mobile and active throughout your day doing errands and housework definitely counts as movement! In fact, if you find yourself at all disabled by your condition, simple everyday tasks such as loading

EXERCISE ASSESSMENT

This is a checklist to help you determine if the exercise routine you are engaged in may be negatively impacting your health. Check off all of the statements that apply to you, tally your score, and see your result below.

- ☐ I am sore the same day of the exercise.
- ☐ I am sore the day after the exercise.
- ☐ I am sore for more than a day after the exercise.
- ☐ I feel exhausted or like I need a nap later in the day following exercise.
- ☐ I can't do certain activities after the exercise.
- ☐ I find that I have a hard time getting motivated to do the exercise.
- ☐ I have a hard time getting through the exercise because of pain or fatigue.

- ☐ I find myself tired or sore during the exercise.
- ☐ I frequently find myself getting injured as a result of exercise.
- ☐ I find the same level of workout getting more difficult, not easier.
- ☐ I find that the exercise causes flares of my autoimmune disease.
- ☐ I get shaky or light-headed in the middle of or immediately following the exercise.

SCORING: Any score higher than 1 or 2 may mean that your currently chosen activity is too intense or depleting for your needs, and you may consider transitioning into a type of activity that is more gentle. Sometimes, a less-intense exercise is optimal long-term, or you may find yourself being able to increase intensity over time.

the dishwasher or working in your garden can be a considerable workout. Others may outsource some of this work to a cleaning company, nanny, or other family members to give them more time to work (most often at that desk job!). Don't underestimate the impact that being active at home can have on your movement needs. Often, these activities can serve multiple goals—creating a clean living environment, preparing healing foods, or playing with children or pets.

EVERYDAY ACTIVITIES THAT KEEP YOU MOVING

- Doing housework
- Cooking
- Gardening
- Walking your dog
- Walking your kids to school
- Walking/cycling to work
- Running errands
- Playing with children
- Shopping
- Doing home improvements

THE BENEFITS OF WALKING

A discussion about types of movement best for those with chronic illness is not complete without giving some extra attention to walking—we believe it can be the best exercise for those with autoimmune disease and chronic illness. The structure of our bodies is designed to enable bipedal movement, or being on our feet (as opposed to sitting). Still need some convincing why walking is an optimal activity? Check out the list below.

- **IT'S MODERATE IMPACT.** Walking is lower impact than running, but not so low that it doesn't provide much benefit in building bone density, like cycling or swimming.

- **IT'S SIMILAR TO HOW OUR ANCESTORS MOVED.** They spent their time working on their feet, walking, and gathering foods. Our bodies are adapted to this type of movement, yet most of us spend more time sitting than standing or walking.

- **IT DOUBLES AS A STRESS-REDUCTION EXERCISE.** Walking can be relaxing, especially when you make an effort to be mindful of your surroundings. Since most of us with autoimmune disease are struggling to manage our stress, we need all the help we can get!

- **IT EXPOSES US TO SUNLIGHT, FRESH AIR, AND NATURE.** All of these components help regulate our immune systems and manage our stress (see Chapter 5).

- **IT CAN BE AN ACTIVITY THAT BUILDS COMMUNITY.** Walking can be enjoyed with others and is a great alternate activity to going out for a meal or drink with friends (especially when you are in the elimination phase!).

- **IT TAKES MINIMAL INVESTMENT.** The only thing you need is a good pair of shoes! No expensive gym, trainer, or fancy equipment is necessary.

- **IT KEEPS US HAPPY.** Studies show that a regular walking routine helps keep depression and anxiety at bay.

- **IT IS GOOD FOR LYMPHATIC FLOW**. Although the lymphatic system has lots of vessels, it lacks a pump and is dependent on movement for lymph flow and drainage.

- **IT CAN BE SCALED TO YOUR NEEDS**. You can walk the block in your neighborhood or try a hike on a more challenging path.

- **IT CAN BE DONE ANYWHERE**. The possibilities are endless—walk close to where you live, in a nearby nature preserve, on the beach, or in a shopping mall.

It is surprising, given all of the evidence in favor of walking, that most people don't seek it out or even consider it exercise. Getting started with a walking routine is simple—just get a good pair of shoes that fit you well and provide the support you need, and you are on your way! Aim to take short walks initially, even starting with 5 to 10 minutes, and then build up to an hour or more per day. You can rotate walking alone mindfully, listening to music or a podcast, or with a buddy—changing up the scenery keeps boredom at bay. Your routine can be as little or as much as your body allows; the key is just to get out there and do it!

Movement Solutions for the Workplace

Many people find it difficult to get the amount of movement they need when they work a traditional desk job, sitting in front of a computer or being in an office every day. Unfortunately, studies show that a 30- to 60-minute workout before or after work does not "undo" the stress caused to the body by sitting. Try some of these suggestions to help mitigate the toll that working a desk job can take on your body.

- **CONSIDER A NONTRADITIONAL DESK**. Treadmill desks, standing desks, and modular (combination) desks are all alternatives to the traditional desk and can be helpful solutions. More important than which type of desk you choose is that you are changing your position throughout the day. Chronic standing can be as detrimental as chronic sitting, so the best solution often includes a variety of options to change it up periodically.

- **TAKE FREQUENT BREAKS**. At least a few minutes every hour, make sure to get up, walk around, and do some simple stretching. You will be amazed at the improvement in your muscle tension, fatigue, mental clarity, and energy levels when you prioritize these movement breaks, no matter how busy or stressful your day at work is.

- **SWITCH UP YOUR CHAIR**. Having a yoga ball handy to replace your regular chair occasionally can help you remember to sit up straight and engage your core as you work. You could also try other options like a kneeling chair.

- **WALK OR BIKE TO WORK AND DURING BREAKS**. If possible, walk or bike to work and try to use some of your break time to get on your feet and move around! Enlist a coworker so you have a buddy to keep you on track.

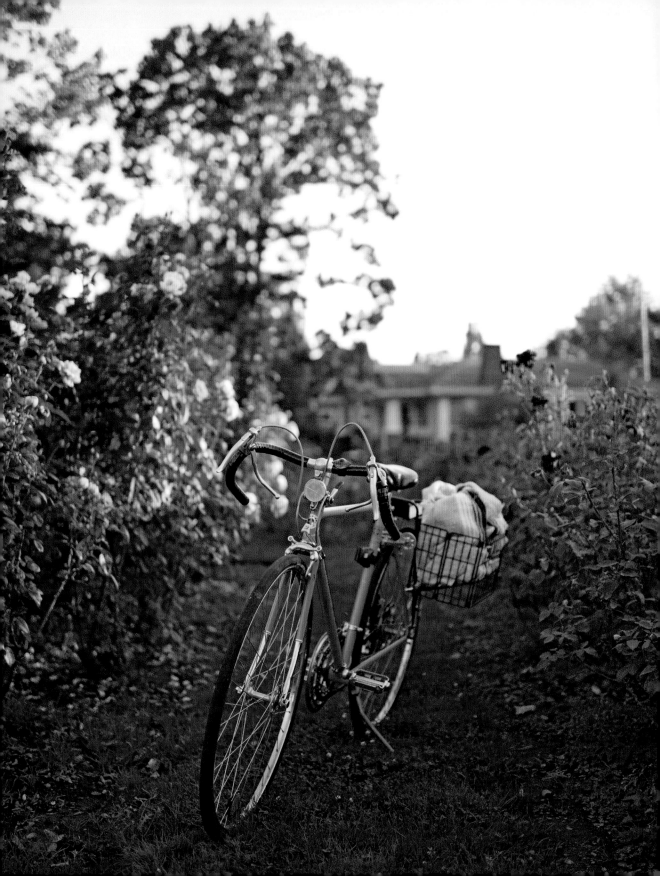

FINDING BALANCE WITH MOVEMENT

Just as your needs in other areas (like sleep and stress management) change over time, your movement needs and abilities are also likely to ebb and flow. It is important to take stock of your current stress level, your physical capabilities, whether or not your autoimmune symptoms are flaring up, and your general resilience at any given time. Constant evaluation and adjustment allow you to take advantage of times when your health is particularly robust and dial back when energy needs to be diverted to healing.

Living well with autoimmune disease means being flexible when your body calls for rest. After a period of strength, it is easy to experience profound disappointment and frustration if physical capability is again limited due to your disease or an unexpected illness. There's no shame in demonstrating versatility in response to those needs.

CALL TO ACTION

We are created for movement. From our powerful brains sending the millions of imperceptible signals required, all the way to our very bones supporting the whole endeavor, literally every fiber is designed for the often undervalued miracle of movement. Fitness of both body and mind cannot be maintained without appropriate physical activity. It is up to us to take advantage of our extraordinary bodies and learn to *move* them in the best ways.

In this chapter, we explored why moving matters and how too much or too little of it, especially for those with autoimmune disease, can be detrimental. The tools outlined here can help you fine-tune your body's movement needs and hopefully discover ideas for getting active. We've placed special emphasis on walking as an ideal fitness routine for autoimmune disease, because it requires almost nothing to start and can easily be scaled to your unique needs. It is a surprisingly simple and empowering step on the autoimmune wellness journey. As British historian G.M. Trevelyan said, "I have two doctors, my left leg and my right."

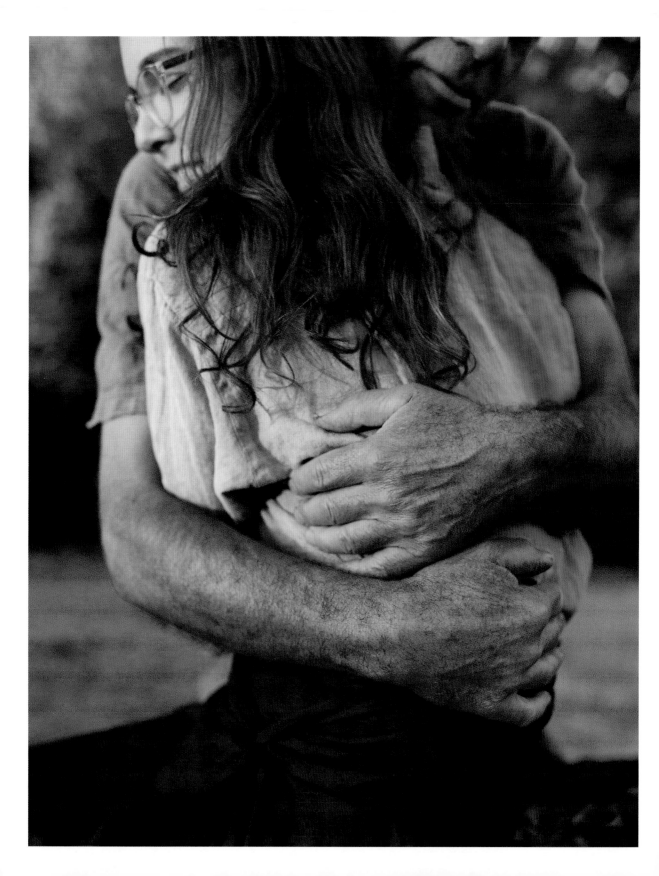

CHAPTER 7

Connect

"Alone and without love, we die. Life itself is as dependent on relationships with others as it is on food." —M. N. BECK

THERE ARE TWO AREAS IN LIFE in which connection is essential in order to gain and maintain our best health—other humans and the natural world. We are not separate from each other, or from our environment. We've divided this chapter into two sections, one devoted to each, so that you can learn about and explore cultivating these connections.

CONNECTING WITH PEOPLE

We have all experienced the hurt from the loss of connection to others, whether it is through death or some other circumstance. Many are surprised to learn that our brains experience this type of emotional pain *just like* physical pain. The very same region of our brains responsible for processing physical pain is also responsible for processing social pain. It is no wonder losing a loved one or a breakup is often described as "being kicked in the gut," or "being broken-hearted." Our brains experience it that way! Neuroscientist Matthew Lieberman, PhD, wrote about this finding in his 2013 book, *Social: Why Our Brains Are Wired to Connect.* It wasn't just that the brain saw these two kinds of pain the same way—the two kinds of pain can even be managed the same way. Further research by Dr. Lieberman showed that Tylenol could dull social pain in much the same way as it dulls physical pain. Why does it matter that our brains group physical and social pain together? It demonstrates on an extremely basic level that our connection with other human beings is fundamental to our health. It's so vital that our brains register both large and small threats to that connection as literally painful events. It's simple! Our need for connection to other human beings, a strong social support network, is a must for good health, just like nourishing food.

ROBUST SUPPORT NETWORKS AND ACHIEVING WELLNESS

Our brains see the loss of connection with other people just like the loss of a limb—both events are registered as pain. It's not just avoiding pain that makes adequate social support important, as there's even more evidence that social support matters to our health. One study revealed that smoking up to 15 cigarettes a day predicted less about your likely survival than a lack of social support. (We are not encouraging you to go pick up a pack here!) Our positive relationships with others have been shown to lower cortisol, the stress hormone we talked about, and increase oxytocin, a hormone responsible for stimulating our sense of calm and connection. Beyond that, it's no secret that lonely, isolated people experience greater levels of stress and depression, both of which carry numerous negative health consequences of their own. We need others not just to avoid pain, but to mitigate health risks and encourage wellness.

Being happy and healthy is not a solitary pursuit. This is even more accurate if you are struggling with autoimmune disease. The ups and downs of chronic illness require us to bravely reveal our vulnerability and find others whom we can rely on for help and support. You are more likely to make the dietary and lifestyle changes we advocate in this book successfully within a loving, caring community. Do not underestimate how significant that network is when it comes to healing and achieving wellness.

Find your tribe and ask them to show up for you as you undertake this journey!

BUILDING A SUPPORT NETWORK

We know intuitively, through countless studies, loads of epidemiological data, and laboratory testing, that a strong support network matters greatly to good health. Even so, at one time or another, all of us may encounter a period where our network is inadequate. Maybe you've just moved far from home, or you've become a new parent, or you're tackling a specific issue that your existing network isn't familiar with—there are many reasons for needing to improve the depth or width of your support network.

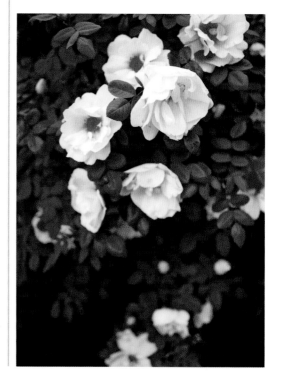

SUPPORT NETWORK EVALUATION

Your support network is the entire community of people around you who value you and help provide for your physical and emotional needs. This network usually operates under "mutual obligation." In other words, you both give and receive support. The four main types of support are emotional, practical, sharing points of view, and sharing information. Having both depth (a few very close, intimate people) and width (a large number of casual friends and professionals) in your network provides a sense of security, belonging, and buffering against the stresses of life.

If you often have the sense that your support network is not strong enough or are wondering if you'll have adequate support as you undertake the autoimmune wellness journey, it can be helpful to evaluate it. The following questionnaire can help you determine if you have a robust support system or if you should take proactive steps to improve it. Give yourself one point for every box that applies to you and tally your score at the bottom.

☐ When I am in need, there are people there for me.

☐ I get the support I need from my family.

☐ I share my ups and downs and receive comfort from a few key people.

☐ I get the support I need from my friendships.

☐ There are key people in my life who treat my needs and feelings as important.

☐ I can count on my friends and family to help me make decisions and work through problems.

☐ I have personal and professional contacts that I can rely on to help me with practical problems (like fixing an appliance).

☐ I have people in my life who are proud of me.

☐ There are several people I can talk to when I am feeling lonely or depressed.

☐ I have someone in my life with whom I feel comfortable sharing intimate personal problems.

☐ I regularly spend time with my family and friends.

☐ I have friends who are there for me, even when it's not fun (like an early morning trip to the airport or packing up a moving van).

☐ There are others in my life who come to me for practical help and support.

☐ If I were in need of caretaking, there are people in my life who would help fill the gaps.

☐ There are people in my life whom I trust and who see me as trustworthy.

☐ I have people in my life who honor important events (like birthdays).

☐ I have people in my life who would be there for me in the event of a crisis.

SCORING: Any score lower than 12 means that you may need to prioritize strengthening your support network. The following sections give you some ideas about how to achieve that.

Nobody ever says, "Geez, I just have way too many caring people in my life who are willing to help me out!"

If you find yourself needing to boost your connections with others, here are some tips on building that support.

- **TAKE RISKS.** There is no opportunity to meet new people and possibly develop rewarding relationships if you don't go for it. Join groups, accept invitations, try new activities, and just generally be open to meeting more people.

- **SPEAK UP.** Unless all your friends and family members are part of a psychic network, they won't know what you need unless you tell them. Learn how to communicate your needs so that those around you can address them.

- **BRANCH OUT.** Use your existing network to form new connections. Ask those around you to introduce you to interesting, fun people they know and who they think you might enjoy getting to know, too.

- **LET GO.** There might be a few relationships in your circle that aren't very healthy. Identify those relationships and look at ways to break the negative tie or reduce the impact it has on you, so that you are open for healthier connections.

- **MAP IT.** If you aren't even sure what kinds of support you are missing or where you might find that support, sit down and figure it out. For example, if you have lots of practical support, but not much emotional support, looking for a group of folks dealing with the same issues would greatly strengthen your network.

- **CHILL OUT.** We meet numerous people over the course of our lives, but only some of them become part of our network and even fewer become true friends. Forming meaningful connections takes time; don't be impatient.

- **TREASURE IT.** Strong relationships are not one-sided. Be sure you find ways to contribute to your important relationships and tell those special people how much you appreciate them in your life.

MAINTAINING KEY SUPPORT RELATIONSHIPS

You may have a great support network but also recognize that a few important relationships need a little "maintenance." Creating lasting, healthy relationships requires effort. Here are a few ideas on strengthening the key connections in your life so that you can count on them over the long haul.

- **LOVE EQUALS TIME.** Be sure you manage your time in a way that allows you to focus on the important people in your network. Make time to go out with your best friend, play with your child, or have a deep talk with your partner. If you don't make time to nurture these relationships, they will deteriorate.

- **DON'T BE A BULLY OR A WIMP.** Assertiveness is expressing your needs and feelings while respecting others' needs and feelings. It is a way to communicate without being aggressive or passive. Being open and honest helps reduce conflicts and misunderstandings in your relationships.

● **KEEP YOUR EARS OPEN.** One of the most important things that close relationships offer is being heard. Knowing that someone cares about you and is willing to pay attention as you share your joys and sorrows is vital. Be sure you are focused and using good listening skills when you are interacting with your loved ones.

● **GET OUT OF YOUR COMFORT ZONE.** Too much routine can allow important relationships to grow stale. People often grow closer when they are in new, unfamiliar situations together. Take a rock-climbing class with your sister or try learning a new language with your partner. Any big or small change can help you bond more deeply.

● **SAY SORRY AND ACCEPT APOLOGIES.** Admitting mistakes and asking for forgiveness as well as letting go of injuries when sincere apologies are offered make for trusting, enduring relationships. The love you could be pouring into a key connection is robbed by the energy required to wait on saying sorry or hold on to a wrong.

ADDRESSING UNSUPPORTIVE RELATIONSHIPS

It's no secret that relationships with family members and close friends will be impacted by a chronic illness. Most of us in the autoimmune community have dealt with the challenges of relationships that become strained around ongoing health struggles. One psychologist, Marie Hartwell-Walker, EdD, writes that this may happen because our culture does not have methods for acknowledging persistent illness or a continual health crisis, unlike the rituals we have around temporary illness or death. Some people may take it personally if you can no longer go out as often or don't have the energy for activities that were shared before. Others may mistakenly believe your diagnosis is "catching," or some may feel helpless so they stop reaching out at all. Still others may be too involved in their own lives to make time for how you are changing. Surprisingly, seeking wellness through major dietary and lifestyle changes can have similar effects on your relationships. Your changing priorities may be perceived as threatening by some of those close to you. Or they may have strong judgments about the new steps you are taking to deal with your autoimmune disease.

It can be helpful to have some ways to handle unsupportive family or friends, whether you are deep into your autoimmune battle or making empowered new decisions on your way to wellness.

● **GIVE THEM TIME.** For many of us in the autoimmune community, the road to diagnosis is very long, often measured in years. Deciding how to respond to your disease can also be a lengthy process. It may take those close to you just as much time to understand and accept a new version of you. You have been steadily altering your view of yourself from the onset of symptoms, but their view of you has not had to progress at the same pace. Try to patiently give them time.

- **NOT EVERYONE CAN GIVE YOU "COMPLETE" SUPPORT.** Adjust your expectations about how much support the people close to you will be able to provide. There are varying degrees of severity with autoimmune diseases, but for all those dealing with it, an autoimmune disease is life changing. We all want complete love and unconditional support while we learn to manage our chronic illnesses. However, the reality is that the amount and kind of support the people around you will be able to offer will differ. Try to acknowledge the positive support that is offered by each person, allowing it to form a "whole," and let go of your wishes for more "complete" support from everyone.

- **FIND OTHERS WHO "GET IT."** Seek out a community of people going through the same disease challenges or working toward wellness with similar approaches. There is valuable support that comes from interacting with others who understand because of personal experience. That support can help fill gaps.

- **WHAT DOES YOUR GUT SAY?** Being aware of your instincts about the positive or negative energy generated by some people is crucial. If you feel bad about yourself,

slightly depressed, or like interactions are uncomfortably forced when you are around a particular person, it might be time to get to the bottom of why that relationship is so strained. Maybe he is actually experiencing something difficult, too, and you could help. Or maybe he has taken your illness or new lifestyle change personally and needs to be reassured that you still value him.

- **ALWAYS CHOOSE TO RESPECT YOURSELF.** If there are people in your life who are not only unsupportive, but actively sabotaging your efforts to cope with your disease or heal, stand up about the unacceptable treatment. Let them know that if they are unable to understand or offer support, you can accept that, but that you will not accept being actively undermined. Negative relationships can be among the major factors that need to change in a wellness journey. You may reconsider whether or not continuing the relationship is appropriate.

AN AUTOIMMUNE-FRIENDLY SOCIAL LIFE

Having one or more autoimmune diseases does not have to mean the end of your social life. If you're about to undertake the autoimmune wellness journey, never fear! Despite making the big changes we advocate in this book, you can still have a fulfilling social life. Having a chronic illness and seeking healing doesn't mean we're fuddy-duddies! Socializing can and should remain a priority. It cements the connections to others that are so critical to good

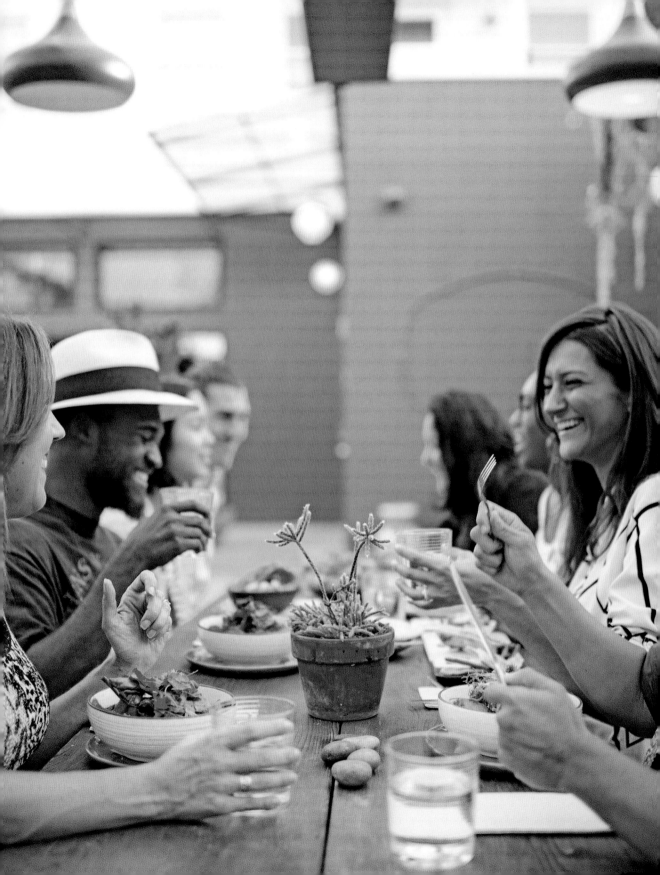

health, and it's just plain fun! Here are some ideas for developing an autoimmune-friendly social life.

- **JOIN A HOBBY GROUP.** Acting, knitting, stamp collecting, birdwatching—the list of options is endless, even if your energy levels need to be conserved.

- **PLAN A DINNER PARTY, POTLUCK, OR PICNIC.** These options allow you to handle the menu or bring your own food, if you have restrictions.

- **MEET FOR TEA, KOMBUCHA, OR FRESH SMOOTHIES.** If coffee at the local shop or a drink at the local bar isn't an option, there are lots of alternatives.

- **GO ON A NATURE WALK OR HIKE.** Nature walks and hikes are great ways to combine connections to nature and people, and you can throw in a resting point, if necessary, to take in the sights and sounds.

- **MAKE AN ART OR CRAFT PROJECT TOGETHER.** There are "paint your own pottery" stores all over the country, or you could grab some supplies and host a "creative juices" party with friends.

- **FIND A CAUSE AND VOLUNTEER.** The research is solid about the health benefits of volunteering, and doing it with others could double the joy of giving.

- **LISTEN TO OR PLAY MUSIC TOGETHER.** Look for opportunities to go see your favorite band with your partner or, if you play, get together with others to jam.

- **MAKE A "LAUGH" DATE.** Laughing is literally good for your health, so plan a funny movie night or go see a live comedy show.

- **JOIN OR START A BOOK CLUB.** Book clubs are one of the easiest, most inexpensive social activities, while also generally being low-key and generating lots of interesting discussion with others.

This list of ideas is just a start—you could do almost any activity you'd like. The real keys to enjoying a great autoimmune-friendly social life are planning and preparation, so your food and rest needs are met before or after activities, clear communication with others so they know what you are capable of handling at any given time, and an open mind about fun in all of its forms.

CULTIVATING BALANCE

We've talked about balance in relation to diet in Chapter 3—learning to walk the line between food as medicine versus food as fear is an important part of this process. We also touched on the idea of balance in managing stress and finding an ideal amount of movement. Why do we come back to this topic so often? It all comes down to homeostasis. Homeostasis is the self-regulating process that biological systems use to maintain stability. Our bodies are ceaselessly working to achieve this in order to keep our systems running smoothly. We see balance as integral to the autoimmune wellness journey because it is integral to existence.

When we speak about balance in this chapter, we mean finding a way to acknowledge your autoimmune disease and honor the battle your body is fighting, while not allowing illness to become your identity. We are also referring to the place where you can be empowered by your wellness journey without letting it dominate your life. Illness as an identity, or healing as your one and only interest, closes you off from connection with others. Without these connections, your life is out of balance.

How you personally will achieve this balance will be unique to you. Each of us must struggle with this aspect of illness and healing on our own. In terms of moving away from illness as your identity, it can be helpful to try viewing the supposed disadvantages of the disease through another lens. Perhaps making a paradigm shift, a change in assumptions, will allow you to recognize positive things that have come into your life as a result of illness. Maybe you've become more resilient, or you have a sharper sense of humor. Similarly, illness can provide perspective on what you want to achieve in life.

When it comes to our interests being dominated by the pursuit of healing, it can help to remember that the whole reason for healing is to use that renewed energy to expand, rather than contract, your life. Reminding yourself that your methods of healing aren't yardsticks for measuring every other aspect of life helps you maintain balance. Even we, with careers in this field and autoimmune diseases of our own, don't spend every minute of every day on these topics.

Colin Wright, an author and international speaker, said, "Extremes are easy. Strive for balance." We agree. Balance—homeostasis—takes work to achieve, but it is best for you and your connections to those you love.

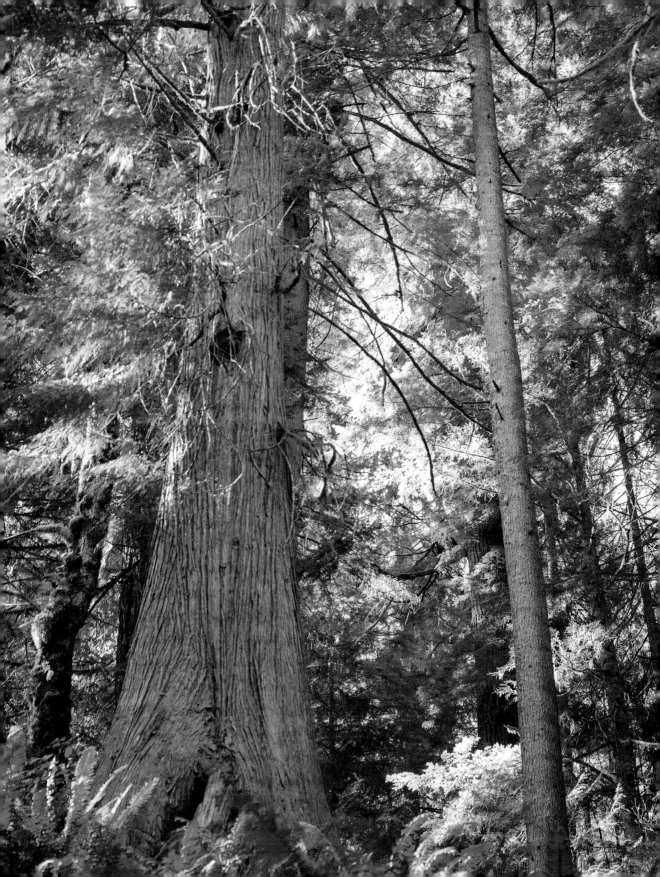

CONNECTING WITH NATURE

"Study nature, love nature, stay close to nature. It will never fail you."
—Frank Lloyd Wright

The relationship between human beings and the natural world runs deep due to our hunter-gatherer past—before cities emerged, we considered the natural world home. Humans have always had to have a relationship with nature, whether that was experiencing or dealing with the elements, cultivating the land, traveling, or using nature to create and develop a higher quality of life. This natural world has provided us with richness in its resources and opportunities, as well as hardship and difficulties due to its unpredictability and inability to be controlled. As much as civilization and technology have removed many of us from nature, we are still dependent on it to sustain our lives—we cannot live without the sun, soil, wind, and water.

Despite not knowing the exact reason why, humans seem to be biologically drawn to nature. People report feeling more calm, at peace, and relaxed when they are in a natural environment. Research on outdoor exposure and health has shown clear benefits, from lowering stress hormones, blood pressure, and heart rate to increased immune function. One possible reason for these effects is because of how inherently stressful our urban, modern lives can be. It seems innate for us to feel at peace and comforted by the natural world.

How exactly does nature affect us? We experience it through a variety of our senses—especially vision, smell, touch, and sound. When we are in a natural environment, we view the plants, trees, and landscape, and we smell the compounds released by the plants and trees. We also feel the uneven ground beneath our feet or on surfaces, like bark and leaves on trees and plants, and hear the sounds of the wind in the trees and the animals that inhabit the landscape. These senses produce changes in our brains, which have a powerful effect on our emotions as well as our physiology. Nature is a soothing, healing force that can be used to enhance our health and well-being. As naturalist and author John Muir wrote, "Thousands of tired, nerve-shaken, over-civilized people are beginning to find out that going to the mountains is going home. Wilderness is a necessity."

Forest Bathing

SHINRINYOKU, translated as "taking in the forest atmosphere" or "forest bathing," has become a popular health practice in Japan for better relaxation and stress management. It is the most popular formal nature activity aimed at achieving better health practiced around the world. The Forest Agency of the Japanese government introduced the concept of *shinrinyoku* in 1982, and there has since been extensive research into the health benefits of such a practice. After isolating individual elements, researchers have postulated that these health benefits come from exposure to the odors of nature, the sounds of streams and animals, and views of the forest scenery, both individually but, more profoundly, when experienced together with other people.

This research indicates that even short exposures to nature can provide the following health benefits.

- Increased physical activity
- Lower levels of depression
- Increased sleep quality
- Regulated immune function
- Improved mood and emotional health
- Lowered cortisol and other stress hormones
- Lowered blood pressure and heart rate
- Increased parasympathetic activity (associated with relaxation and less stress)
- Lowered sympathetic activity (associated with stress states)
- Better recovery from stress

The Japanese are aware of these health benefits and encourage their citizens to engage in this practice in an effort to elevate public health. The news of positive study results has spread the practice worldwide. How do you do it? Just simply find yourself a forest where you can be in nature, either sitting or walking to take in the scenery. You may like to meditate or practice mindfulness, take a stroll, or enjoy a picnic with a friend. It's that easy!

Duration of Exposure

The Japanese research on *shinrinyoku* indicates that even a short duration of time spent in the forest (1 to 3 hours) can produce beneficial physiological as well as emotional changes. It is definitely worthwhile to consider getting some exposure to nature a few times a week, if not daily. If you set yourself up right, this can double as another health-promoting activity like exercise, stress reduction, or connecting with a close friend or family member. It could be as simple as taking your morning walk at a local nature preserve or park instead of on the treadmill at the gym!

Although many studies have shown benefit from short durations of time spent in the forest, a 2009 study found that a weekend camping trip produced increased immune function. The part of the immune system that was boosted was the NK cells, those that are integral in detecting and eliminating cancer cells as well as pathogens. The best part was that not only did the participants have a large increase in immune function when they returned but also they continued to show a boost over a month after the trip was over! A similar study compared a weekend vacation in a city versus a natural setting, with accommodations, activity, and food all the same as a control. The participants who spent the downtime in an urban environment got no boost in immunity, while those vacationing in a natural, tree-filled setting had a positive effect. Making an effort to be in nature for an extended period of time can certainly help you live healthier, even if you are only able to do it occasionally.

Connection to Other Aspects of Health

Being in nature is very closely connected to two other aspects of health, movement and stress reduction. It can also have a profound impact on a third, sleep quality. A 2014 study in Finland showed that people had a greater sense of well-being and better sleep quality when exercising the same amount in nature as opposed to indoors—one reason to get your movement outside as opposed to at the gym! Incorporating time in nature with some other health-promoting activities can help you maximize your efficiency while prioritizing your healing. For instance, taking a walk in the forest with a good friend helps you manage your stress, move your body, connect socially, sleep better, and connect with nature—kill five birds with one stone!

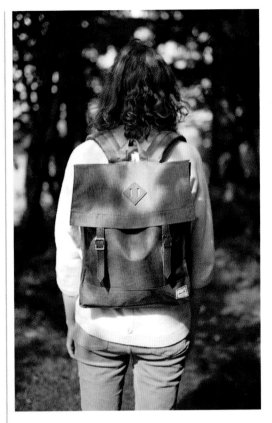

What about Your Indoor Environment?

In modern life, it is almost impossible to get away from spending time indoors, and you should consider optimizing your indoor environment as well as getting out in nature. Biophilic design is that which incorporates connection to the outdoors in an indoor environment, through natural ventilation and materials, natural lighting, outdoor views, landscaping, and interior designs that mimic nature. While research has been focused mostly on the workplace, studies show that indoor plants are correlated with higher productivity, a reduction in indoor air pollution, and improved moods.

The Japanese have done extensive research about isolating forest qualities and reproducing their beneficial effects indoors, like the use of essential oils or natural wood surfaces. One study found that having a room paneled in 45 percent natural wood produced similar effects on stress reduction, and yet another found that inhaling the essential oils of cedar or cypress produced a similar effect. If it is necessary for you to spend a lot of time indoors, it may be prudent to consider some

I've always been a lover of the outdoors, and it became difficult to remain connected to nature while I was in the depths of my autoimmune crisis. In those days, I attempted to get outside once a day, and even though I lived in an urban environment, grounding my feet in the small patch of grass in my backyard, listening to the birds, and feeling the breeze on my skin always energized me. I also cultivated a lot of houseplants, which kept my indoor space bright and lively even when I couldn't make it outdoors. When the weather was nice, I would eat outside as much as possible and work in the yard growing lettuce and herbs. As I gained strength, my short neighborhood walks were able to take me to my local arboretum for a more immersive experience. I discovered that being in nature is so healing to me that I have since left the city and moved to a more rural environment. Although, in those beginning stages, there were many barriers to connecting with nature (illness, weather, living in an urban environment), making it a part of my routine helped nourish my spirit and manage my stress, and it is a habit I continue to cultivate today.

of these findings when designing or decorating your home or workspace.

How to Start Connecting with Nature

Cultivating a connection with nature is something that is a process—start with some small changes like taking your lunch break in a nearby park or walking a few times a week in a nature preserve. As you reawaken that connection, you may find yourself seeking deeper experiences with the natural environment like the occasional camping trip or cabin vacation. The best way to connect is to find the way that feels good to you—for instance, it might be best for you to lie down and listen to the sounds of nature instead of taking a strenuous hike. Any effort you can make to include nature into your routine on a regular basis, especially in combination with the other aspects of a healthy lifestyle

(such as movement, stress management, or community), will benefit your healing process. Here are some ideas for how to get started.

- **FIND YOUR LOCAL GREEN AND OPEN SPACE AND USE IT OFTEN!** You likely have a park or open space walking distance from your home or work that can be used for exercise, relaxation, or enjoying a meal with friends or family, even if you live in an urban area. Make an effort to visit this space as often as possible, weather permitting, in order to reap the benefits of maintaining that constant connection to nature.

- **FIND YOUR LOCAL NATURE PRESERVE OR HIKING TRAILS.** Ideally, this is a location that is still easily accessible (within 20 to 30 minutes from your home or work) but provides you with a larger and more natural environment than a local park for longer walks and to provide minimal distractions.

MAKE YOUR INDOOR ENVIRONMENT MORE NATURAL. Use houseplants to green up your indoor environment and clean your air! Large windows that let in plenty of natural light as well as greenery and nature from outside can also help. Diffuse essential oils found in the forest (like cedar or cypress) to simulate the experience.

PLAN FREQUENT NATURE DAY TRIPS. Try to get out in nature for a longer period of time, say 2 to 3 hours at least once a week. Some ideas are as follows:

- Plan an outdoor picnic.
- Play a game or sport at the park.
- Go for a long walk in a nature preserve.
- Take a hike on a local trail.

PLAN SOME EXTENDED TIME IN NATURE. Depending on how adventurous you are, you can plan to "rough it" for a weekend or longer. Some may prefer lodging with a kitchen, especially when complex dietary needs are considered. Whatever accommodations you decide on, the important part is the immersion in nature as well as disconnection from technology and the pace of modern life. Plan to do this at least once or twice per year. Some ideas are as follows:

- Backpacking
- Car camping
- Glamping (luxury camping)
- RV camping
- Vacationing in a cabin

CONSIDER LIVING WHERE NATURE IS MORE ACCESSIBLE. This is not a change that is possible for everyone, but the next time you are looking for a new living situation, consider its accessibility to local parks, open space, hiking trails, nature preserves, and national parks.

CALL TO ACTION

In this chapter, we looked at the importance of connection, to people and to nature. Our interdependence on others and the natural environment is so obvious but very often overlooked. This is especially true when it comes to their importance to our health. It is so easy to dismiss how much a hug or sunlight matters, but the truth is that none of us would have made it, healthy and whole, from infancy to now without them. Understanding the significance of connection to others and nature, evaluating the strength of those connections, and learning ways to enhance both your support networks and your links to the natural world are steps that will pay dividends on your wellness journey. Although we presented it last, we believe taking time to connect is essential, not just an afterthought. Author Bryant McGill sums it up: "There is a deep interconnectedness of all life on earth, from the tiniest organisms, to the largest ecosystems, and absolutely between each person." We cannot be healthy without connection.

CHAPTER 8

Recipes + Meal Plan

YOU'VE FINALLY ARRIVED AT THE FUN part of the book—our collection of nutrient-dense anti-inflammatory recipes! All of these recipes are compliant with the elimination phase of the Autoimmune Protocol and avoid grains, legumes, dairy, eggs, nuts, seeds, and nightshade-family vegetables and spices. Better yet, they include healing foods that contain powerful nutrition aimed at restoring health and strengthening your body! As you learned in Chapter 3, there is a wide spectrum of possible dietary interventions for those with autoimmune disease. Whether your goal is just to start eating gluten-free or to dive in with the elimination phase, this chapter will serve as an incredible resource for you.

If you are new to cooking for yourself, short on time or energy, or want to maximize your time spent in the kitchen, you are in luck—these recipes are simple to execute, don't contain a lot of hard-to-find ingredients, and store well in the refrigerator or freezer to help you get ahead of the curve. Most of them are one-pot, making cleanup a breeze. We know how living with autoimmune disease can zap your energy, and cooking yourself wholesome meals should not be just another drain! Best of all, these recipes will keep the rest of the family happy, too, whether or not they eat a restricted diet. If you are just getting your feet wet (see the Slow-and-Steady Transition Guide on page 74) or jumping in right away (see the Cold-Turkey Transition Guide on page 72), you will find something of value here. In addition to the recipes, you'll find a 4-Week Meal Plan at the end of the chapter, complete with shopping lists, tool lists, pantry basics, and a guide on selecting food. Let's get cooking!

A note about breakfast: You'll notice that the recipes included here are a far departure from what is common on the standard American diet. Choose to nourish yourself with a complete, nutritious meal, even if it comes in the form of soup for breakfast. Even though this way of life isn't familiar, other cultures have been enjoying it for centuries!

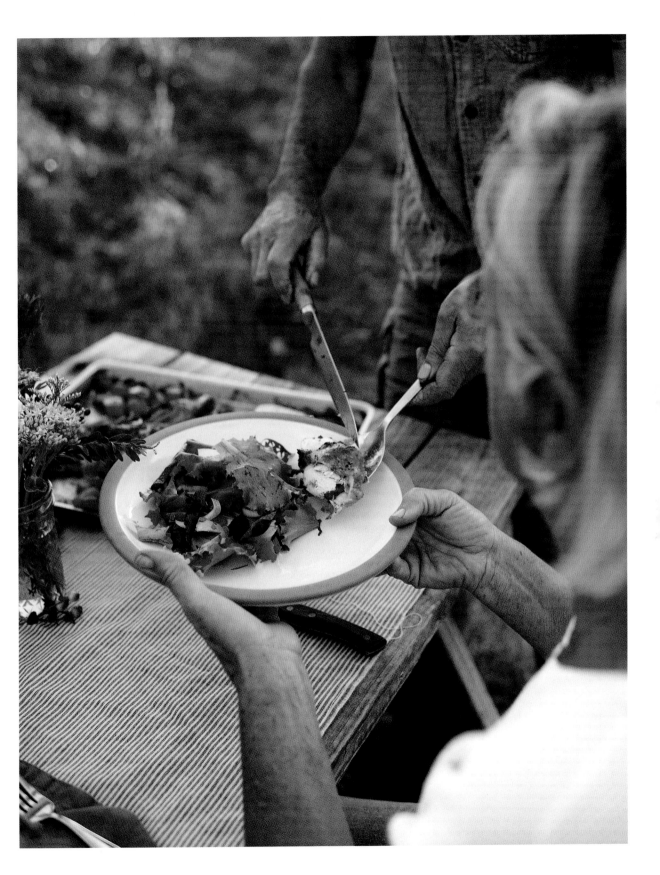

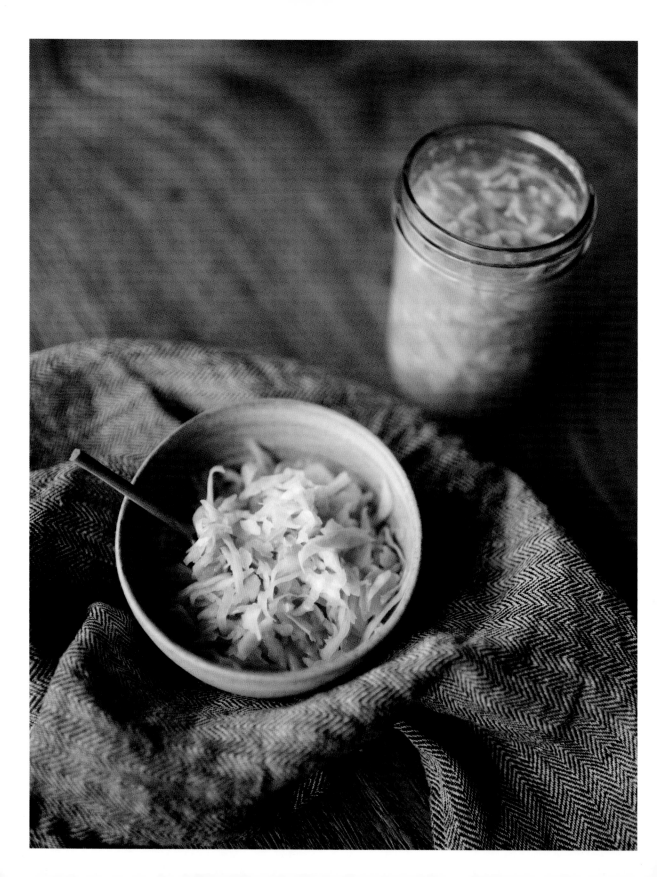

Recipes

BONE BROTH

TIME: 8 TO 24 HOURS
MAKES: 3 to 4 QUARTS

4   **quarts filtered water**

2   **(or more) pounds bones
from a good source
(knuckle and marrow bones
work well, but you can use
any type)**

2   **tablespoons apple cider
vinegar**

1   **bay leaf**

STOVETOP METHOD

1 Place all ingredients in a large stockpot or slow-cooker and bring to a boil. Lower the heat so the water is barely simmering; cover.

2 Occasionally skim the surface for any scum that may appear during cooking.

3 Cook for at least 8 hours and up to 24 hours, being sure to check periodically to ensure that the broth is still at a bare simmer. The longer you cook the bones, the more rich and nutritious the broth will be.

PRESSURE COOKER METHOD

1 Place all ingredients in a pressure cooker, making sure not to exceed the fill line. Lock the lid and place over high heat until the cooker comes to high pressure, then turn down to the lowest setting that will maintain this pressure (you may need to use a flame tamer).

2 Let the broth cook for 3 hours, then turn off the heat and let the broth depressurize and cool naturally.

WHEN THE BROTH IS FINISHED (USING EITHER METHOD)

Let cool, then strain and portion the broth into containers for storage. After the liquid is strained, pick through any bones that are still intact and save them to add to the next batch, tossing those that fell apart. (You can usually get a few batches out of larger beef knuckle bones, while chicken bones last only for 1 or 2 batches). You can refreeze used bones if you are not ready to make another batch of broth immediately.

STORAGE: Keeps for a week in the refrigerator. Also freezes well.

The Autoimmune Wellness Handbook

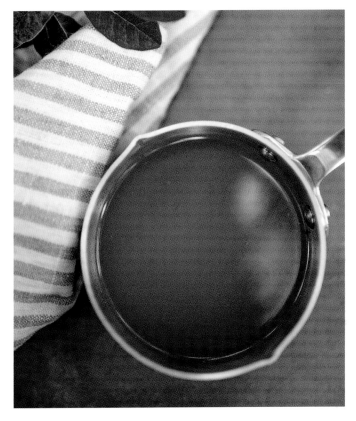

VARIATION: There are many ways to vary bone broth, such as browning the bones in the oven before cooking or adding some herbs and spices or vegetables while it is cooking. We like to avoid salting the broth so that it doesn't impact the amount of salt used in the recipes. The broth can also be boiled to reduce so that it is concentrated and stores more easily. As you continue to make broth, you will get into a flow, and can make it according to your preference.

SOURCING: Bones should not be expensive or difficult to find. The best source is a farmer you trust, maybe at a farmers' market or through a community supported agriculture program. If you don't have those sources available to you, a lot of natural-food stores sell bones from grass-fed meat—be sure to ask the butcher if you don't see any available! Also, you can start a bag in your freezer for storing any bones from the meat you consume. Just toss them into the bag, and freeze to make broth at a later time. Feel free to use any type of bones, even if they have been previously cooked, to make broth—beef, lamb, chicken, and turkey all work well (it is okay to combine types). If you'd like to purchase already-made bone broth, check out Resources on page 261.

RENDERED ANIMAL FAT

TIME: 2 TO 4 HOURS
MAKES: ABOUT 2 CUPS

1 **pound animal fat, cold (lard, tallow, duck fat, or suet works well)**

¼ **cup water**

1 Cut the fat into small pieces—ideally smaller than 1 inch. Place them in a large cast-iron pot or a slow-cooker with the water and turn the heat to the lowest setting.

2 Let the fat cook on low for an hour or so, stirring every so often.

3 Once there is a considerable amount of fat melted (maybe a third to a half of the solid fat), strain most of it through a fine-mesh strainer into another pot and set aside to cool, leaving about ¼ cup in with the solid fat and set aside. Place the remaining unrendered fat back on the stove. Continue doing this until there are just solids and no unrendered fat left.

4 Once all of the fat is in the second pot and warm enough to be liquefied but not still hot, transfer into a glass jar for storage.

STORAGE: Keeps for a few months in the refrigerator. Also freezes well.

NOTE: You can take the solids (the cracklings) left in the pot after the rendering process and bake them for 20 minutes at 400°F. (This might also produce some extra rendered fat!) They make a great crunchy snack or salad topping.

SOURCING: Make sure to use fat from healthy animals—those that have been raised on pasture and fed an appropriate diet. These are likely to have the best fatty acid profile and nutrition. You can either save bits of fat cut off from larger pieces of meat to render or get fat from your butcher. See Resources on page 261 for sourcing animal fat or purchasing it already rendered.

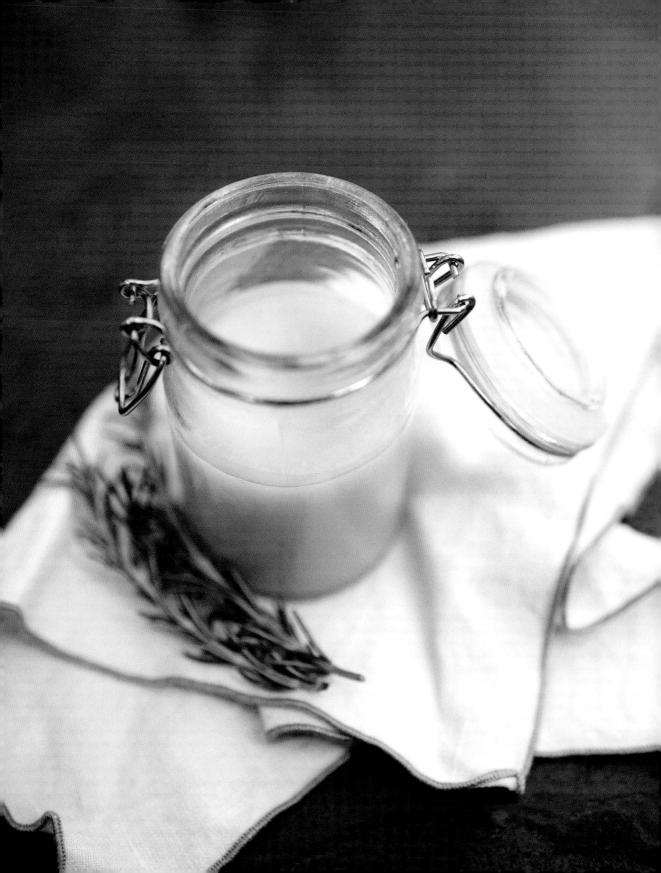

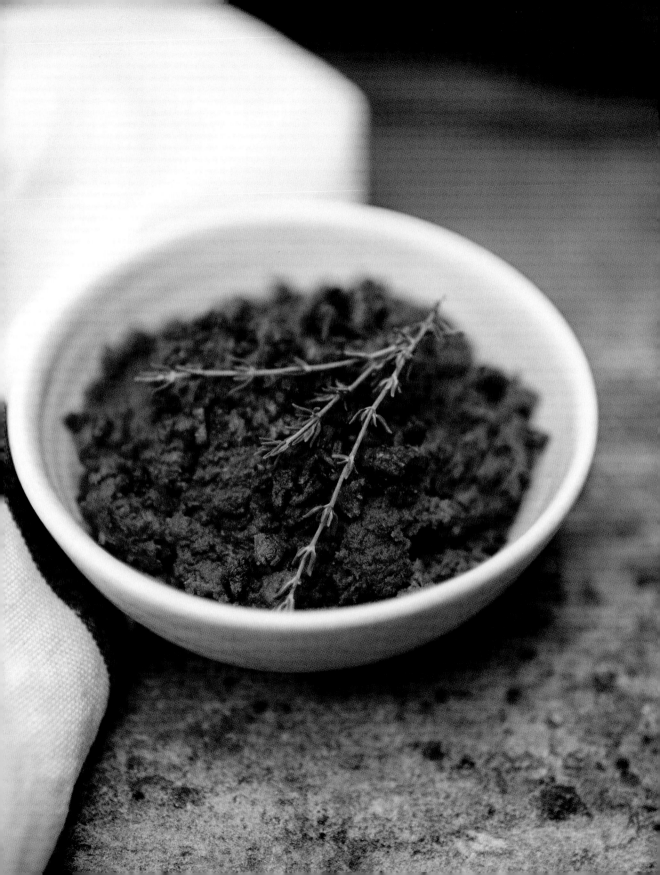

BACON—BEEF LIVER PÂTÉ WITH ROSEMARY AND THYME

TIME: 35 MINUTES
MAKES: ABOUT 2 CUPS

1 Cook the bacon slices over medium heat in a cast-iron skillet, flipping as needed. Cook until crispy. Transfer to a paper towel–lined plate to cool, reserving the fat in the pan.

2 Add the onions and cook on medium-high heat for about 5 minutes, stirring. Add the garlic and cook for a minute, then add the liver, rosemary, and thyme. Cook for 2 to 5 minutes per side, or until the liver is no longer pink in the center. Set aside to cool for a few minutes.

3 Transfer the mixture into a blender or food processor with the coconut oil and sea salt. Process until it forms a thick paste.

4 Place the pâté into a small bowl. Chop the cooled bacon into the bowl in fine pieces and combine.

5 Garnish with the fresh herbs and serve with vegetable slices.

STORAGE: Keeps in the refrigerator for several days. Also freezes well.

NOTE: This recipe is difficult to make in a standard blender; you really need a high-powered machine with a tamper for best results. Alternately, you could use a food processor.

6   slices bacon (check ingredients to ensure it is gluten- and nightshade-free)

1   small onion, minced

4   cloves garlic, minced

1   pound grass-fed beef liver, rinsed, dried, and sliced into 2- to 3-inch pieces

2   tablespoons minced fresh rosemary

2   tablespoons minced fresh thyme

⅓   cup coconut oil, melted

½   teaspoon sea salt

    Fresh herbs, for garnish

    Carrot or cucumber slices, for serving

FERMENTED VEGETABLES

TIME: 20 MINUTES, PLUS 2 TO 3 WEEKS FOR FERMENTATION
MAKES: 2 QUARTS

4–5 pounds cabbage
(about 2 heads)

2 tablespoons sea salt,
or more if needed

YOU ALSO NEED

2 (1-quart) glass jars with
airlocks

Tamper (optional)

Clean fermenting weights
or stones

1 Finely shred the cabbage and place it in a bowl in batches, sprinkling each batch with a layer of sea salt. When you are finished with the shredding, use your hands to massage the cabbage well until it breaks down and becomes soft (about 10 minutes). Let it sit for 10 minutes to release its juices.

2 Pack the cabbage very tightly into jars, pushing all of it down until it is completely submerged by its own juices (a tamper is helpful here). Leave about 1½ inches of head space, and add some additional brine (made by dissolving 1 teaspoon sea salt in 1 cup water) if there is not enough liquid to fully submerge the cabbage. Place fermenting stones on top to weigh down the cabbage, tighten the lid and ensure the airlock is installed properly (refer to the instructions that came with your unit, as they can vary). It is possible to ferment without an airlock, just be sure all of the cabbage is submerged, and check it often to make sure it isn't spoiled.

3 Let the cabbage ferment at room temperature for 2 to 3 weeks; during this time, the vegetables will bubble a little and intensify in flavor. If any scum appears, remove it with a spoon. Taste it starting at 2 weeks, and when the taste is to your liking, you can remove the airlock and weights, put a regular lid on the jars, and store in the refrigerator.

STORAGE: Fermented vegetables will keep for a few months in the refrigerator.

VARIATIONS: The possibilities for varying your fermented vegetables are endless—you can use different types of cabbage, carrots, beets, garlic, ginger, and many other vegetables in different combinations to make a rich array of tasty probiotic foods. Check Resources on page 261 for links to great websites dedicated to fermentation.

GELATIN GUMMIES

1 To make one of the flavor options, begin by combining the fruit juices in a small saucepan and sprinkling the gelatin on top. Do not stir. Set aside for 5 to 10 minutes, until the gelatin has "bloomed" or absorbed all of the liquid.

2 Meanwhile, add the honey (and ginger, if making Citrus-Ginger option) to a small bowl with a pour spout.

3 When the gelatin has bloomed, place it on the stove and turn on the heat to the lowest setting. Heat for 30 seconds to 2 minutes, stirring constantly with a whisk, until completely liquid and the gelatin has dissolved. Be careful here, as you do not want the liquid to simmer or get hotter than it needs to—this will cause the gummies to stink.

4 Immediately pour the gelatin mixture into the container with the honey and stir to combine. Pour into silicone molds or the bottom of a small roasting dish.

5 Let chill for 8 hours in the refrigerator. If you used molds, place them in the freezer for 5 minutes; this will make them release more easily. If you elected not to use molds, slice into 1-inch squares and serve.

STORAGE: Keeps for a week or two in the refrigerator; do not freeze.

NOTE: Look for high-quality, grass-fed gelatin online from either Great Lakes or Vital Proteins and gummy molds at various online retailers (see Resources on page 261).

VARIATION: This recipe tastes great with various fruit juices, although those that are more concentrated and tart (cranberry, for example) taste best. Pineapple juice won't work because it has enzymes that break down the gelatin.

TIME: 15 MINUTES, PLUS 8 HOURS TO SET
MAKES: 2 TO 3 DOZEN

POMEGRANATE

- 1½ cups pomegranate juice
- 2 lemons, juiced
- ⅓ cup grass-fed gelatin
- ¼ cup raw honey

BLUEBERRY

- 1½ cups blueberry juice/extract
- 2 lemons, juiced
- ⅓ cup grass-fed gelatin
- ¼ cup raw honey

CITRUS-GINGER

- 1 cup orange juice (from 3–4 oranges)
- ½ cup lemon juice (from 6–8 lemons)
- ⅓ cup grass-fed gelatin
- ¼ cup raw honey
- 1 teaspoon ground ginger

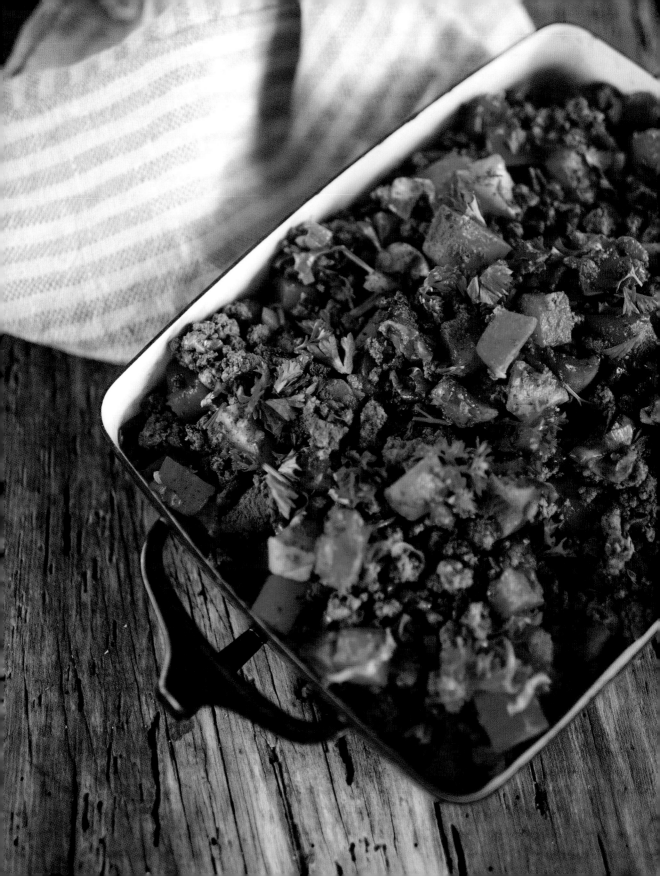

BUTTERNUT BREAKFAST BAKE

1 Preheat the oven to 400°F.

2 Brown the ground beef in a heavy-bottomed skillet on medium-high heat, making sure to stir occasionally to ensure even browning. When the beef is fully cooked, spoon into a large bowl, reserving the juices in the pan.

3 Turn the heat to medium and, in the same pan with the reserved juices, sauté the leeks until tender, about 4 minutes. Add 1 teaspoon of the cinnamon, the salt, cloves, and ginger and stir to combine, cooking just until fragrant.

4 Add the leek mixture, squash, apples, and coconut oil to the bowl with the beef, and stir to combine. Pour into a 9 by 13-inch baking dish, cover tightly with foil, and bake for 45 to 50 minutes, or until the squash is tender.

5 Remove the foil and sprinkle with the remaining teaspoon of cinnamon and the parsley.

STORAGE: Keeps for a week in the refrigerator. Also freezes well.

VARIATION: If you can't get your hands on butternut squash, feel free to use a different variety (like acorn), or substitute sweet potatoes.

TIME: 1 HOUR, 20 MINUTES
SERVES: 4 TO 6

1½ pounds grass-fed ground beef

3 leeks, white and light green parts only, chopped

2 teaspoons ground cinnamon, divided

1 teaspoon sea salt

½ teaspoon ground cloves

½ teaspoon ground ginger

1 butternut squash, peeled and cut into 1½-inch chunks (about 4 cups)

2 sweet apples, cored and chopped (about 2 cups)

¼ cup coconut oil, melted

3 tablespoons chopped fresh parsley

NUTRIVORE'S BREAKFAST

TIME: 1 HOUR, 15 MINUTES
SERVES: 6 TO 8

VEGETABLES

2　large sweet potatoes, cut into 1½-inch chunks (about 6 cups)

2　tablespoons solid cooking fat (page 170), melted

½　teaspoon sea salt

1　bunch of kale, stems removed and finely shredded

PATTIES

2　pounds grass-fed ground beef

¼　cup grass-fed beef liver, ground or grated (see Notes)

1　tablespoon minced fresh oregano

1　tablespoon minced fresh rosemary

1　tablespoon minced fresh thyme

1　teaspoon sea salt

½　teaspoon garlic powder

¼　teaspoon onion powder

1 Preheat the oven to 400°F.

2 Place the sweet potatoes in a large bowl with the cooking fat and sea salt, and stir to combine. Transfer to a baking dish and place in the oven, cooking for 30 minutes and being sure to stir once or twice.

3 While the sweet potatoes are cooking, add all of the patty ingredients to a large bowl and combine using your hands. Form into 6 to 8 patties, place on a plate, and set aside. If you are prepping the uncooked patties to cook later, place them in a storage container separated with slices of wax paper and place them in the refrigerator for storage.

4 When you are ready to cook the patties, place a skillet on medium heat. When it is hot, add the patties to the pan, and cook for 10 minutes, flipping once or twice, until cooked through.

5 Add the kale to the sweet potatoes and stir to combine. Place back in the oven and cook for another 5 minutes, or until the sweet potatoes are soft. Serve each patty on a bed of kale and sweet potatoes.

STORAGE: Prepped patties keep for 3 to 4 days in the refrigerator; cooked patties keep for 5 to 6 days, and the vegetables keep for a week.

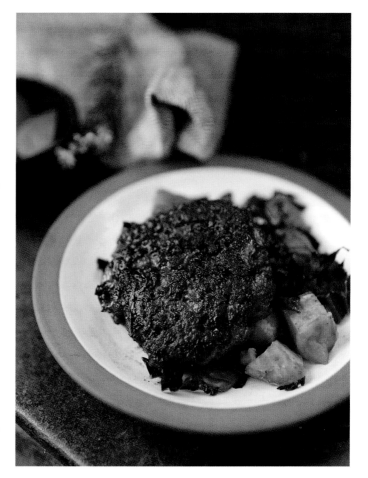

NOTES: If you are going to batch-cook this recipe, it is best to prep the patties and cook them fresh as you eat them (it only takes 10 minutes in the morning!). If you need them to last longer than a few days, you will want to cook them before storing in the refrigerator or freezing. We find that they taste best when cooked fresh.

Instead of preparing the liver every time we make this recipe, we like to have some grated or shredded liver already frozen and ready to go. Take a chunk of frozen liver and either use the shredder blade on your food processor or a box grater to process it, and then freeze in ½-pound batches to add to the patties or other recipes like our Hidden Liver Chili (page 189).

GREEN BREAKFAST SOUP

TIME: 2 HOURS, 30 MINUTES
SERVES: 8 TO 10

1   **large, whole pastured chicken (5–6 pounds)**

1   **bay leaf**

1   **tablespoon apple cider vinegar**

1   **tablespoon sea salt + additional, to taste**

2   **tablespoons solid cooking fat (page 170)**

1   **onion, chopped**

4   **cloves garlic, minced**

1/3   **cup peeled and minced fresh ginger (3- to 4-inch piece)**

2   **large sweet potatoes, chopped into 1 1/2-inch chunks (about 6 cups)**

2   **large zucchini, chopped into 1 1/2-inch chunks (about 2 cups)**

1   **bunch Swiss chard, stems and leaves divided and chopped**

2   **cups button mushrooms, thinly sliced**

1   **bunch green onions (ends removed), thinly sliced, for serving**

1   **lemon, cut into wedges, for serving**

1 Begin by cleaning the chicken (rinse it under cold water and remove loose bits of fat and other tissue). Place it in a large stockpot. If it doesn't fit, you will have to cut it into halves or quarters (kitchen shears help here—start by cutting up one side of the backbone).

2 Add the bay leaf, vinegar, and 1 tablespoon sea salt. Fill the pot with cold water until the chicken is just covered. Bring to a boil, and then cover tightly and lower the heat to a bare simmer. Cook until the meat is tender and falling off the bone, 60 to 90 minutes—the lower the simmer, the more tender the chicken will come out. Skim the surface of the broth to remove any scum that may appear during cooking.

3 Remove the chicken from the pot and set aside to cool. Pour the broth through a fine-mesh strainer, being careful to save the broth in another pot! Discard the bay leaf.

4 Place the empty pot back on the stove, add the solid cooking fat, and turn the heat to medium. When the fat has melted and the pan is hot, add the onions and cook, stirring, for 7 minutes, or until translucent. Add the garlic and ginger and cook, stirring, for another few minutes, until fragrant.

5 While the onions are cooking, remove the meat from the chicken carcass, shred it with two forks (CAUTION: hot!), and set it aside in a bowl. Keep the bones to add to your next batch of Bone Broth (page 168).

6 Add the sweet potatoes and broth back to the pot, bring to a boil, and then cover and turn down to a simmer. Cook for 10 minutes.

7 Add the zucchini, chard stems, and mushrooms, and cook for another 5 minutes, or until the vegetables are tender. Turn off the heat and stir in the chard leaves.

8 Carefully transfer half of the soup to a blender, blend for 30 seconds, and transfer back to the pot. Alternately, you could use an immersion blender to blend about half of the vegetables. (CAUTION: Make sure you have a blender that can handle hot liquid, and make sure to use a towel above the lid to protect your hands from getting burned.)

9 Return the blended liquid to the soup pot, with the chicken. Add salt to taste.

10 Serve each bowl garnished with green onions and a squeeze of fresh lemon juice.

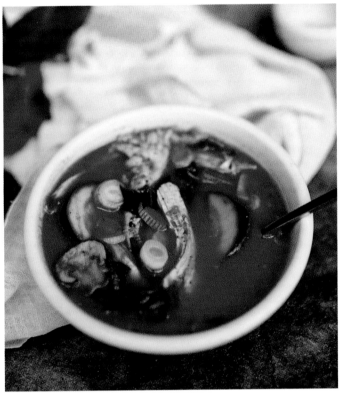

STORAGE: Keeps for a week in the refrigerator. Also freezes well.

NOTE: Depending on the size of chicken you have, this recipe may take a fairly large (7- to 8-quart) soup pot. If yours isn't that large, you will want to use a smaller chicken (2 to 3 pounds) and scale down the sweet potatoes.

DOUBLE PORK PESTO PATTIES WITH WILTED CHARD

**TIME: 25 MINUTES
SERVES: 4**

1 cup packed basil

⅓ cup olive oil

1 teaspoon lemon juice

1 clove garlic, minced

1 pound pastured ground pork

4 slices bacon, minced (check ingredients to ensure it is gluten- and nightshade-free)

2 large bunches rainbow chard, tough stems removed, leaves cut into long ribbons

Salt, to taste

1 Place the basil, olive oil, lemon juice, and garlic in a blender or food processor and process on high until smooth. Set aside.

2 Place the ground pork and bacon in a large bowl, add the basil mixture, and combine all ingredients by hand. Form 4 large patties.

3 Preheat a heavy-bottomed skillet on medium-high heat. When the pan is hot, add the patties and cook for 5 to 7 minutes per side, until completely cooked through. Remove and set aside, reserving the juices in the pan.

4 Turn the heat down to medium, and add the chard to the skillet. Don't worry if it doesn't all fit initially—you can continue to add chard as it wilts. Cook, stirring, until the chard is wilted and the liquid evaporates, 7 to 8 minutes. Season with salt.

STORAGE: Prepped, uncooked patties keep for 3 to 4 days in the fridge; cooked patties keep for 5 to 6 days, and the wilted chard keeps for about 2 days. Freeze between slices of wax paper for long-term storage.

NOTE: If you are following this recipe as a part of the meal plan, cook the patties as written but halve the chard portion, using only one bunch of chard. Cook the second bunch fresh on the third day—it only takes a few minutes!

The Autoimmune Wellness Handbook

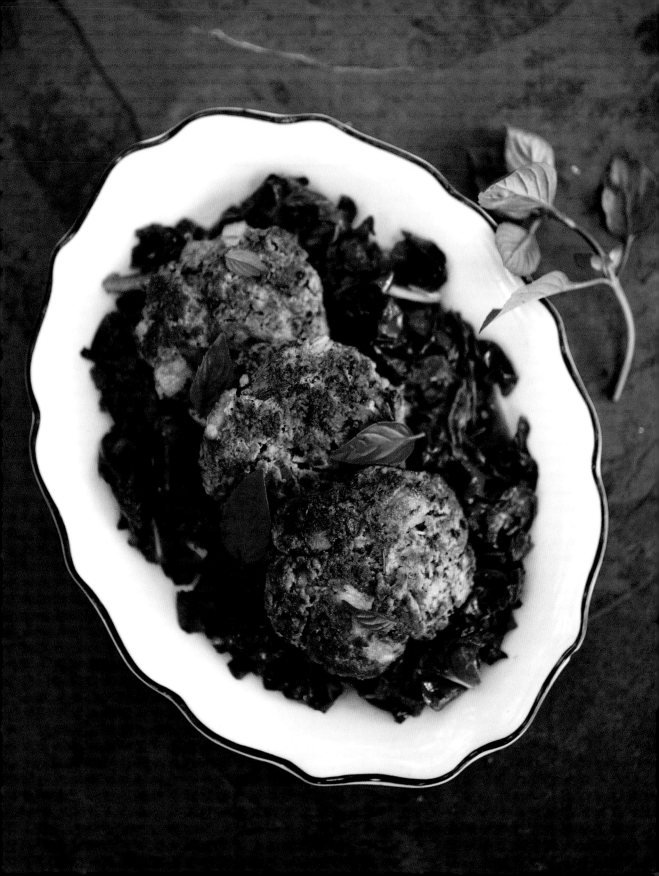

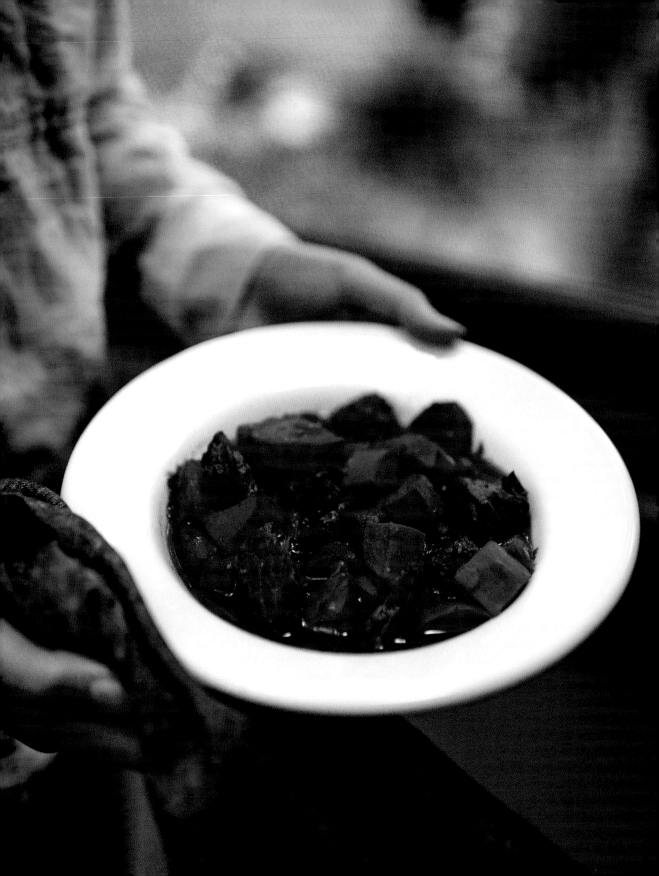

BALSAMIC BEEF STEW

1 Place the meat in a small bowl and coat with the salt. Heat the solid cooking fat in a heavy-bottomed skillet on medium-high heat. When the fat has melted and the pan is hot, add the stew meat. Cook for 5 minutes, turning occasionally for even browning. Place the browned meat in the bottom of a slow-cooker or pressure cooker.

2 Turn the heat down to medium and add the onions to the skillet, cooking for 7 minutes, until translucent. Add the garlic and thyme, and sauté for another couple of minutes, until fragrant. Turn off the heat and add to the meat in the slow-cooker or pressure cooker.

3 Add the sweet potatoes, carrots, celery, and 1 cup of the broth to the meat mixture and cook on low for 8 hours or high for 4 hours, if using a slow-cooker. Alternately, cook for 35 minutes under high pressure using a pressure cooker.

4 Add the remaining ½ cup broth, the vinegar, and coconut oil to the skillet used for the onion mixture. Bring to a boil, turn down to a simmer and reduce by half. Place in the refrigerator as the stew cooks.

5 When the stew is finished cooking, stir in the vinegar mixture and serve hot.

STORAGE: Keeps for a week in the refrigerator. Also freezes well.

NOTE: Use a refined coconut oil for this recipe to avoid an overly strong coconut flavor.

TIME: 50 MINUTES TO 8 HOURS, DEPENDING ON COOKING METHOD
SERVES: 6

1½	pounds grass-fed beef stew meat
1	tablespoon sea salt
2	tablespoons solid cooking fat (page 170)
1	onion, chopped
3	cloves garlic, minced
1	tablespoon minced fresh thyme
2	large sweet potatoes, peeled and chopped (about 6 cups)
6	carrots, peeled and chopped (about 3 cups)
2	ribs celery, chopped (about 1 cup)
1½	cups Bone Broth (see recipe on page 168)
½	cup balsamic vinegar
2	tablespoons coconut oil

THAI SEAFOOD CHOWDER

TIME: 40 MINUTES
SERVES: 6

6 cups Bone Broth (see recipe on page 168)

1 piece (1-inch) fresh ginger, peeled and grated

1 lime, zested (zest reserved) and cut into wedges

4 cloves garlic, minced

1 tablespoon sea salt

2 white sweet potatoes, peeled and cut into 1¹/₂-inch chunks (about 4 cups)

1 tablespoon solid cooking fat (page 170)

2 cups shiitake mushrooms, sliced (use button mushrooms if you can't find them)

1 bunch green onions (ends removed), chopped

1 large head of bok choy, chopped

1 pound shrimp, peeled, deveined, and tails removed

¹/₂ pound firm white fish (like cod or halibut), chopped

1 (14-ounce) can full-fat coconut milk (check ingredients to ensure no thickeners or additives)

1 cup packed basil, chopped

1 Combine the broth, ginger, lime zest, garlic, sea salt, and sweet potatoes in a large, heavy-bottomed pot. Bring to a boil, reduce to a simmer, and cook for 12 minutes, uncovered.

2 Meanwhile, heat the solid cooking fat in a heavy-bottomed skillet on medium heat. When the fat has melted and the pan is hot, add the mushrooms and green onions. Sauté until the mushrooms are tender, about 4 minutes. Stir the mushroom mixture and bok choy into the broth mixture.

3 Stir in the shrimp, fish, and coconut milk. Bring back to a simmer and cook for another few minutes, until the shrimp and fish are cooked through and appear opaque.

4 Serve with basil and lime wedges.

STORAGE: Keeps for a few days in the refrigerator.

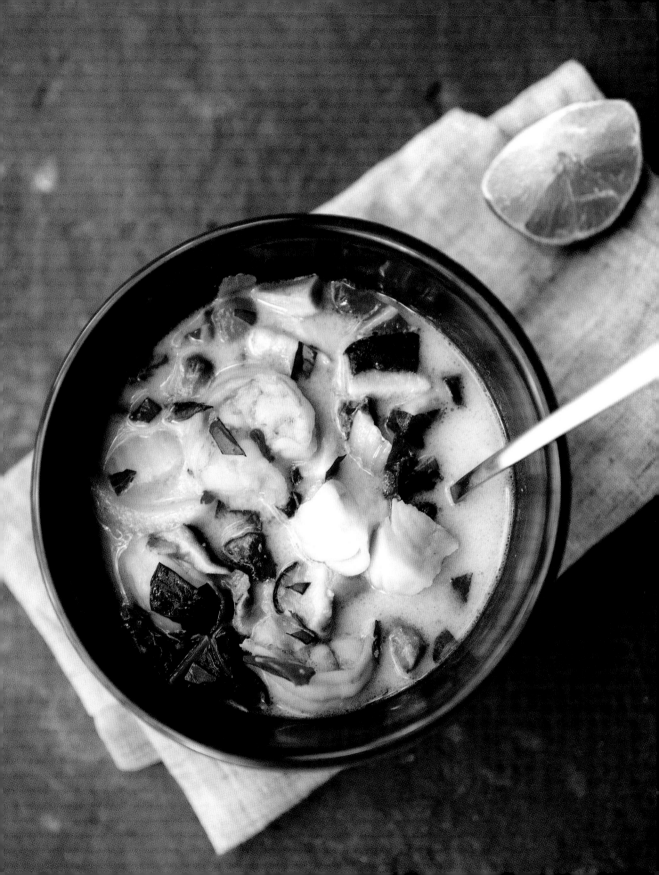

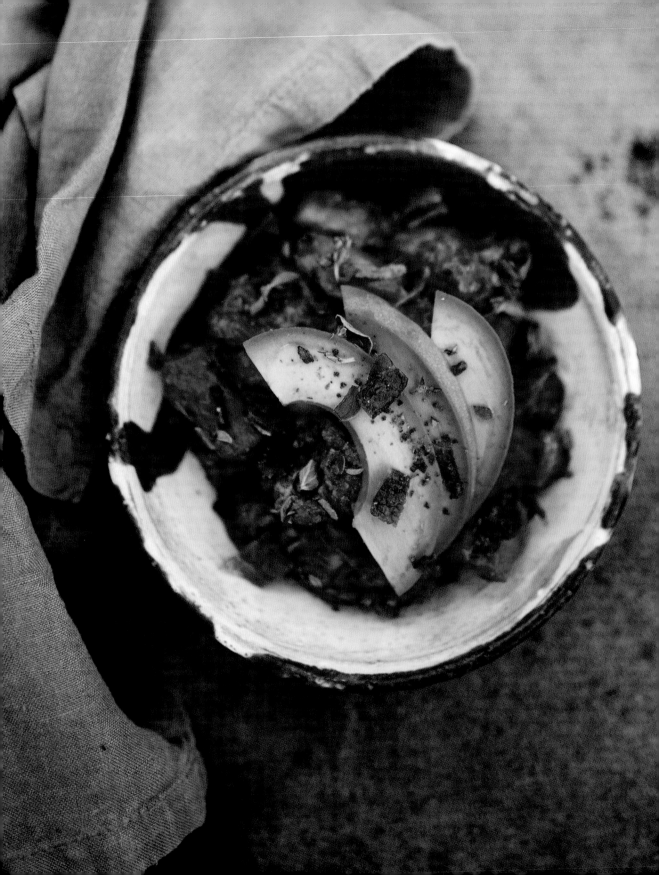

HIDDEN LIVER CHILI

1 Add the slices of bacon to a large heavy-bottomed pot on medium heat, and cook, turning when necessary, until crispy, about 10 minutes. Set aside to cool. Crumble, leaving the fat in the pan.

2 Add the onion to the pan and cook for 5 to 7 minutes, stirring, until translucent. Add the garlic and cook another 3 minutes, until fragrant.

3 Add the bone broth, sea salt, parsnips, carrots, celery, and oregano to the pot, bring to a boil, and turn down to a simmer. Cook, covered, for 20 minutes.

4 Meanwhile, brown the ground beef in a skillet on medium-high heat, being sure to stir it occasionally so that the meat is browned evenly.

5 Add the pumpkin, ground beef, and liver to the pot with the vegetables and cook for another 10 minutes, until the vegetables are tender.

6 Add the lemon juice and fresh ginger, and serve garnished with avocado slices and crumbled bacon.

STORAGE: Keeps for a week in the refrigerator, without the avocado. Also freezes well.

NOTE: Instead of preparing the liver every time we make this recipe, we like to have some grated or shredded liver already frozen and ready to go. Take a chunk of frozen liver and either use the shredder blade on the food processor or a box grater to process it, and then freeze in ½-pound batches to add to this chili.

TIME: 1 HOUR, 15 MINUTES
SERVES: 6

3–4 slices bacon (check ingredients to ensure it is gluten- and nightshade-free)

1 yellow onion, chopped

4 cloves garlic, minced

2 cups Bone Broth (see recipe on page 168)

1 teaspoon sea salt

3 parsnips, cut into 1½-inch chunks

2 carrots, chopped

4 ribs celery, chopped

¼ cup fresh oregano, minced

2 pounds grass-fed ground beef

2 (15-ounce) cans pumpkin puree (check ingredients to ensure no thickeners or additives)

½ pound grass-fed beef liver, ground or grated (see Note)

1 lemon, juiced

1½ tablespoons grated fresh ginger

Avocado slices, for garnish

LEMONGRASS-SCENTED CHICKEN STEW

TIME: 2 HOURS
SERVES: 8

1   large, whole pastured chicken (5–6 pounds)

1   bay leaf

4   stalks lemongrass

2   tablespoons solid cooking fat (page 170)

1   onion, chopped

1   piece (2 inches) fresh ginger, peeled and minced

1   piece (2 inches) fresh turmeric, peeled and minced

1   large butternut squash, peeled, seeded, and cubed (about 6 cups)

1   lemon, juiced

1   teaspoon sea salt

1   bunch cilantro, stems removed and roughly chopped

     Avocado, for garnish (optional)

1 Begin by cleaning the chicken (rinse it under cold water and remove loose bits of fat and other tissue). Place it in a large stockpot. If it doesn't fit, you will have to cut it into halves or quarters (kitchen shears help here—start by cutting up one side of the backbone).

2 Fill the pot with cold water until the chicken is just covered. Add the bay leaf, cover, and bring to a boil, turning down to a bare simmer. Cook until the meat is tender and falling off the bone, 60 to 90 minutes. The lower the simmer, the more tender the chicken will come out. Skim the surface of the broth to remove any scum that may appear during cooking.

3 Meanwhile, slice off the root ends of the lemongrass stalks, as well as the green part 5 to 6 inches from the bottom. Take the flat part of the knife and press down on the lemongrass on the cutting board—this is called bruising and it will help release the oils and flavor the stew. Set aside with the other spices.

4 Remove the chicken from the pot and set it aside. Pour the broth through a fine-mesh strainer, being careful to catch the broth in a second pot! Discard the bay leaf and set the broth aside.

5 Place the empty stockpot back on the stove and heat the cooking fat on medium heat until it is melted and the pot is hot. Add the onions, and cook for about 5 minutes, stirring, until they begin to soften and brown slightly. Add the lemongrass stalks, ginger, and turmeric, and cook for a few more minutes, stirring to ensure that they don't burn.

6 Add the butternut squash, reserved broth, lemon juice, and sea salt to the pot. Bring to a boil and then turn down to a simmer. Cook for 5 minutes.

7 Meanwhile, use two forks to remove the meat from the chicken (CAUTION: hot) and set aside. Keep the bones to add to your next batch of Bone Broth (page 168).

8 Remove the lemongrass stalks from the stew, and add the chicken. Cook for another 5 to 10 minutes, or until the squash is just tender.

9 When the stew is finished, turn off the heat and stir in the cilantro. Serve garnished with fresh avocado, if using.

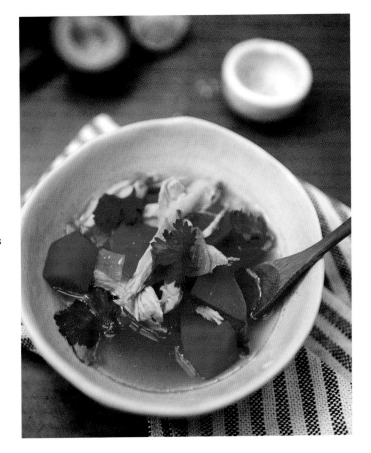

STORAGE: Keeps for a week in the refrigerator; freezes well.

NOTE: Depending on the size of chicken you have, this recipe may take a fairly large (7- or 8-quart) soup pot. If yours isn't that large, you will want to use a smaller chicken (2 to 3 pounds) and scale down the butternut squash.

VARIATIONS: Don't have winter squash? This stew tastes great with carrots, but you will need to extend the cooking time in step 6 to 30 minutes. Don't have fresh ginger or turmeric? Substitute 1 teaspoon dried ginger and 1 teaspoon ground turmeric for fresh. Don't have time to cook the chicken? Use a clean rotisserie or previously cooked chicken and 4 quarts of bone broth and skip steps 1, 2, and 4.

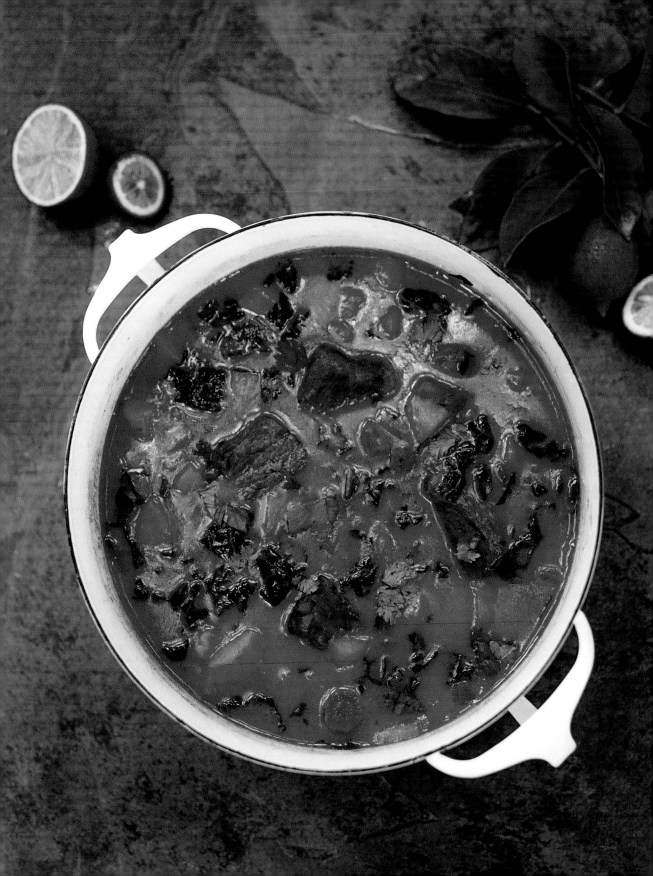

BEEF CURRY SOUP

TIME: 1 HOUR, 45 MINUTES
SERVES: 4

1 Heat the solid cooking fat in a large heavy-bottomed pot on medium-high heat. When the fat has melted and the pan is hot, brown the stew meat for 5 to 7 minutes, stirring once or twice to brown evenly. Remove to a plate and set aside. If your pot is too small to fit all of the stew meat on the bottom without touching, brown in two batches.

2 Turn the heat down to medium and add the onions. Cook for 7 minutes, or until translucent. Add the garlic and ginger and cook for another couple of minutes, stirring, until fragrant.

3 Add the bone broth, water, vinegar, 1 teaspoon sea salt, and browned meat to the pot. Bring to a boil, cover, and then turn down to a bare simmer and cook for 30 minutes. Check to make sure the stew is cooking at a very low simmer and not boiling; this will ensure that the meat stays tender.

4 Add the parsnips, carrots, turmeric, and cinnamon to the pot. Cook at a bare simmer for another 45 minutes, or until the vegetables are just tender.

5 Add the coconut milk and kale to the pot. Continue to cook at a bare simmer for another 10 minutes, being sure to stir a couple times as the kale cooks and reduces in size.

6 Turn off the heat, stir in half of the cilantro and all of the lime juice, and salt, to taste. Serve warm, garnished with the remainder of the cilantro.

STORAGE: Keeps well in the refrigerator for a week. Also freezes well.

VARIATIONS: Can't find parsnips? Use rutabagas or turnips to switch things up! This recipe also works well with alternate greens (like collards or chard) as well as lamb or goat instead of the beef.

2	tablespoons solid cooking fat (page 170)
1½	pounds grass-fed beef stew meat
1	large yellow onion, chopped
3	cloves garlic, minced
1	piece (1½ inches) fresh ginger, peeled and minced
1½	cups Bone Broth (page 168)
½	cup water
1	tablespoon apple cider vinegar
1	teaspoon sea salt + additional to taste
4	large parsnips, chopped into 1½-inch chunks
3	large carrots, chopped
1	tablespoon ground turmeric
⅛	teaspoon ground cinnamon
1	(14-ounce) can full-fat coconut milk (check ingredients to ensure no thickeners or additives)
1	bunch kale, stems removed and chopped
1	bunch cilantro, stems removed and roughly chopped
	Juice from 1 lime

MOROCCAN CHICKEN THIGHS WITH APRICOTS AND OLIVES

**TIME: 1 HOUR, 15 MINUTES
SERVES: 4**

2   tablespoons solid cooking fat (page 170)

2   pounds pastured boneless, skin-on chicken thighs

1   onion, chopped

1   piece (1½ inches) fresh ginger, peeled and minced

3   cloves garlic, minced

3   large carrots, chopped

5   ribs celery, chopped

1   cup Bone Broth (page 168)

½   cup dried apricots, quartered

½   cup green olives, halved (without pimento)

1   lemon, ends trimmed, halved lengthwise, and thinly sliced

¾   teaspoon sea salt

½   teaspoon ground turmeric

¼   teaspoon ground cinnamon

1   tablespoon minced fresh oregano

1 Heat the solid cooking fat in a large heavy-bottomed pot on medium-high heat. When the fat has melted and the pan is hot, add the chicken thighs, skin-side down, cooking on one side for 3 to 5 minutes or until the skin is golden brown and crispy. Don't fuss with them to ensure that they get crispy! Remove from the pan and set aside.

2 Turn the heat down to medium. Add the onions, and cook, stirring, for 5 to 7 minutes, or until translucent. Add the ginger and garlic, and cook, stirring for another couple of minutes, until fragrant. Add the carrots and celery and cook, stirring, for 5 more minutes.

3 Add the bone broth to the pot, along with the apricots, olives, lemon, sea salt, turmeric, and cinnamon. Stir to combine. Add the chicken back to the pot, nesting it into the vegetables and liquid, crispy-skin-side up, and sprinkle with the oregano. It may seem like the pot doesn't have a lot of liquid, but the chicken will soften up and become more juicy as it cooks. Turn down to medium-low, cover, and simmer for 20 minutes. Rearrange the chicken so that it is just nested into the vegetables (there should be more liquid now) and cover and simmer for another 10 minutes, or until the chicken is cooked through.

4 Serve warm.

STORAGE: Keeps in the refrigerator for about a week; also freezes well.

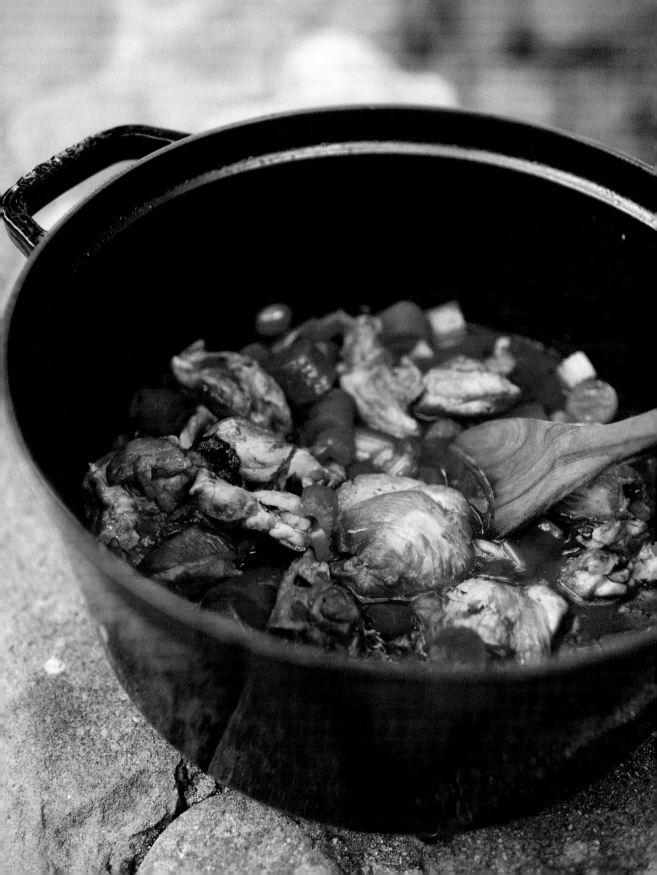

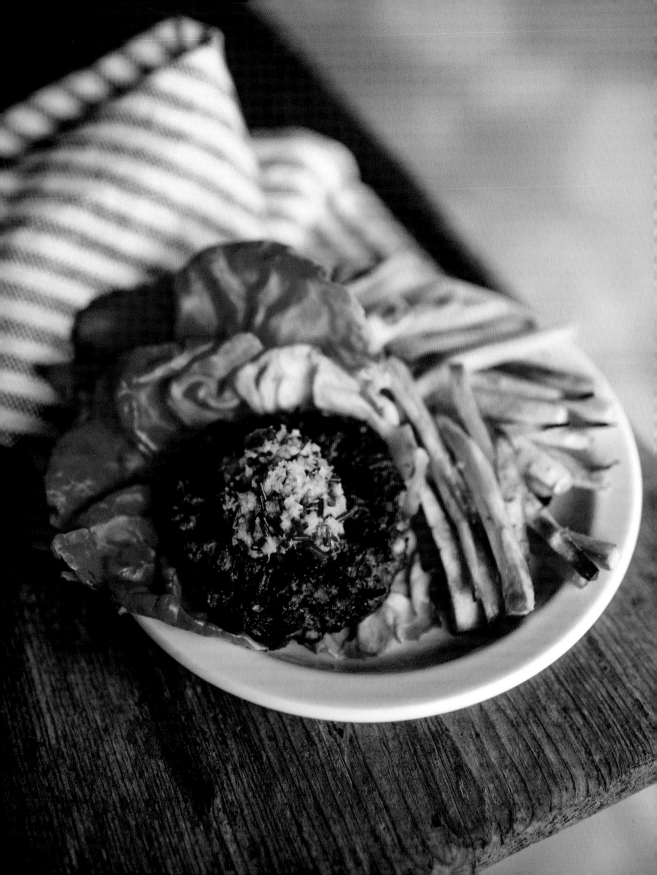

APPLE-BEET BURGERS WITH PARSNIP FRIES AND HORSERADISH SPREAD

1 Preheat the oven to 425°F. Line two baking sheets with parchment paper.

2 Place the parsnips in a large bowl and toss with the salt and fat. Spread evenly on both of the baking sheets, and place in the oven for 25 to 30 minutes to cook, tossing once.

3 While the parsnips are in the oven, combine all of the burger ingredients in a large bowl and mix by hand to combine. Form into 4 large patties.

4 Heat the grill or a heavy-bottomed skillet on medium-high heat. When the grill or pan is hot, cook the patties for 8 minutes per side, or until fully cooked.

5 Combine all of the spread ingredients in a small bowl and whisk together. Set aside.

6 When everything is finished cooking, serve warm with the horseradish spread on top of the burgers.

STORAGE: Patties and parsnips keep for 5 to 6 days; spread keeps for 2 to 3 days.

NOTE: Because of the color of the beets, these burgers may appear undercooked when they are done. When in doubt, use a thermometer to make sure they reach 155°F internally.

TIME: 50 MINUTES
SERVES: 4

FRIES
2	pounds parsnips, peeled and sliced into "fries"
2	tablespoons sea salt
2	tablespoons solid cooking fat (page 170), melted

BURGERS
1	pound grass-fed ground beef
1/2	cup grated beet (about 1 small beet) (see Note)
1/2	cup grated sweet apple (about 1 small apple)
1/4	cup minced white onions
1	teaspoon smoked sea salt
2	teaspoons minced fresh thyme

SPREAD
1/2	cup peeled, grated fresh horseradish
1/4	cup minced fresh chives
1	tablespoon apple cider vinegar
1	teaspoon honey
3	tablespoons olive oil

LAMB TAGINE
WITH CAULIFLOWER "RICE"

TIME: 50 MINUTES TO
8 HOURS, DEPENDING ON
COOKING METHOD
SERVES: 4

1   pound lamb stew meat

1   tablespoon sea salt

4   tablespoons solid cooking
     fat (page 170), divided

1/2 cup dried apricots, halved

1/2 cup prunes, halved

1/2 cup raisins

3/4 cup Bone Broth (page 168)

2   tablespoons apple cider
     vinegar

2   tablespoons lemon juice

1   teaspoon ground cinnamon

1   teaspoon ground ginger

1   teaspoon ground turmeric

1   small red onion, diced

1   head cauliflower, roughly
     chopped

1 Place the stew meat in a small bowl and coat with the salt.

2 Place 2 tablespoons of the solid cooking fat in a heavy-bottomed skillet on medium-high heat. When the fat has melted and the pan is hot, add the stew meat, turning every few minutes to ensure even browning.

3 Place the stew meat and the remaining ingredients, except the cauliflower, into a slow-cooker or pressure cooker. Cook on low for 8 hours or high for 4 hours, if using a slow-cooker. Cook for 35 minutes under high pressure using a pressure cooker.

4 Before the tagine finishes cooking, process the cauliflower in a food processor by pulsing until rice-size granules form. Be careful not to overprocess. Set aside.

5 Place the remaining 2 tablespoons of solid cooking fat in a heavy-bottomed skillet on medium heat. When the fat is melted and the pan is hot, sauté the cauliflower for 5 minutes, stirring, until soft.

6 Serve the tagine over the warm cauliflower.

STORAGE: Keeps for a week in the refrigerator. Freezes well.

Photo shown on page 224.

EMERALD SALMON
WITH ZESTY GREEN SAUCE

TIME: 45 MINUTES
SERVES: 4

1 Preheat the oven to 425°F. Place the broccoli, asparagus, and fennel in a large bowl. Add the coconut oil and ½ teaspoon of the sea salt, and stir until all of the vegetables are coated in oil and salt.

2 Transfer the vegetables to a large rimmed baking tray or dish, making sure they are arranged evenly. Place in the oven and cook for 10 to 12 minutes, or until the vegetables are just softened.

3 Make a space for the salmon in the middle of the baking dish by moving the vegetables to the outside. Place the salmon in the baking dish, sprinkle with the remaining ¼ teaspoon sea salt, and arrange the vegetables around it. Place in the oven and cook for 10 to 15 minutes, or until the thickest part of the salmon is opaque and flakes easily with a fork (the cooking time will vary depending on how thick the fish is).

4 Meanwhile, place all of the sauce ingredients in a blender and blend on high for 30 seconds, until thoroughly combined.

5 Serve the vegetables and salmon warm, drizzled with a generous portion of the green sauce.

STORAGE: Salmon keeps for a couple of days in the refrigerator; vegetables and sauce will keep for a week. Sauce freezes well.

VARIATION: This recipe works great with Brussels sprouts instead of broccoli.

SALMON

1   crown broccoli, chopped into 1½-inch pieces

½   bunch asparagus, stemmed and cut into thirds

1   bulb fennel, chopped into 1½-inch pieces

2   tablespoons coconut oil, melted

¾   teaspoon sea salt, divided

1   pound wild-caught salmon fillet

SAUCE

1   bunch cilantro, stems removed (about 1 cup)

2   cloves garlic, roughly chopped

1   piece (½ inch) ginger, peeled and roughly chopped

⅓   cup olive oil

    Juice and zest of ½ lemon

2   tablespoons water

¼   teaspoon sea salt

CITRUS-GINGER BRINED PORK ROAST

TIME: 4 HOURS, PLUS 6 TO 8 HOURS FOR BRINING
SERVES: 4 TO 6

BRINE

8	cups water, divided
1/2	cup chopped fresh ginger
1/2	cup sea salt
1	tablespoon orange zest
1 1/2	cups orange juice
1	tablespoon apple cider vinegar
2–3	pounds pastured pork roast

RUB

1	tablespoon orange zest
1	tablespoon peeled and grated fresh ginger
3/4	teaspoon thyme
2	cloves garlic, minced

VEGETABLES

1	butternut squash, peeled and chopped into 1 1/2-inch chunks (about 4 cups)
1	pound carrots, peeled and chopped (about 4 cups)
1	cup packed fresh basil
1/3	cup olive oil
2	teaspoons orange juice
2	teaspoons orange zest
1/2	teaspoon sea salt
1	clove garlic, minced

1 To make the brine, boil 4 cups of the water with the ginger. Allow to cool and mix with the remaining brine ingredients (including the remaining water), except the pork roast. Place the roast in a large covered pot (slow-cooker inserts work really well), pour the brine liquid over it, and cover. Place the pot in the refrigerator for 6 to 8 hours (see Note).

2 Drain the roast and discard the brine. Rinse the roast with cool water, pat dry, and place in a roasting pan. Set aside.

3 Preheat the oven to 225°F.

4 Place all of the rub ingredients in a food processor or blender and process for 30 seconds, or until combined. Coat the entire roast in this mixture. Leaving the fat cap facing up, place the roast in the oven to cook for 3 hours, or until the internal temperature reaches 145°F.

5 While the roast is cooking, place the squash and carrots in a large bowl. Process the basil, olive oil, orange juice, orange zest, sea salt, and garlic in a food processor or blender until smooth. Pour over the vegetables and stir to coat. Place the vegetables in a single layer on a baking sheet.

6 When the roast is finished, remove from the oven, tent with foil, and allow to rest for 20 minutes before carving. Turn the oven temperature up to 400°F. Roast the vegetables in the oven for 30 minutes, stirring once halfway through for even browning.

7 Carve the roast as the vegetables finish cooking, and serve together.

STORAGE: Keeps for a week in the refrigerator.

NOTE: Don't exceed 8 hours of brining for this recipe.

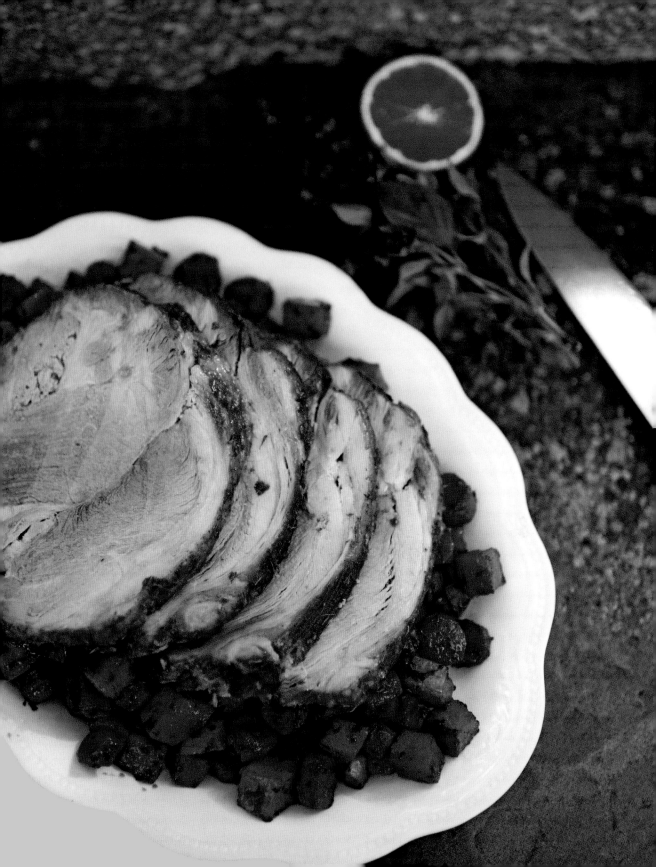

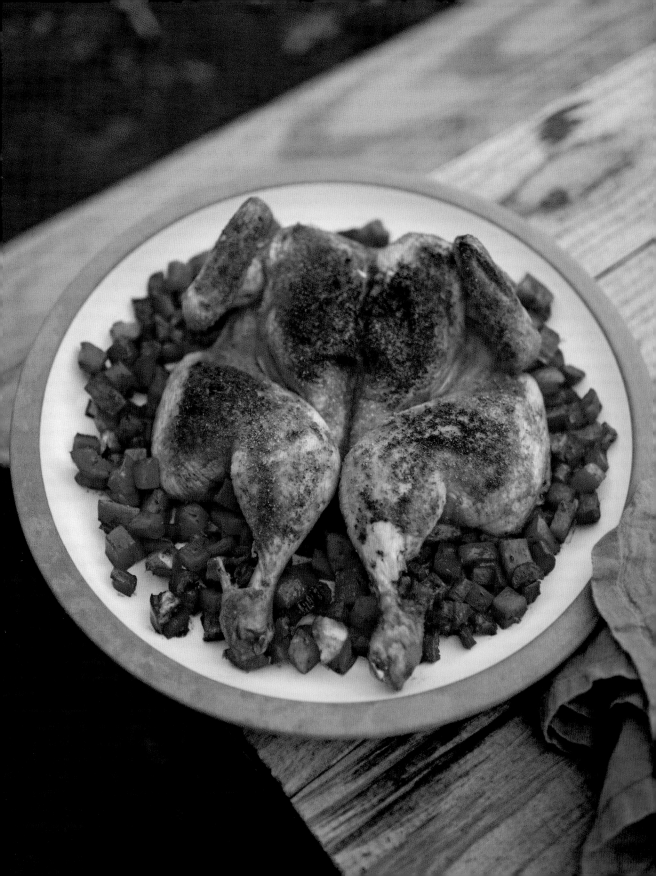

SPATCHCOCKED CHICKEN WITH TURMERIC VEGGIES

TIME: 1 HOUR, 30 MINUTES
SERVES: 4

1 Preheat the oven to 425°F. Place the chopped rutabagas, carrots, and apples into a large mixing bowl. Add the cooking fat, thyme, turmeric, ½ teaspoon of the sea salt, and a pinch of cinnamon, and stir until well combined.

2 Transfer the vegetables to a large rimmed baking tray or dish, making sure they are arranged evenly. Set aside.

3 Rinse the chicken thoroughly under cold water. Place the chicken, breast-side down, in the sink, and using a pair of kitchen shears, cut along the backbone, starting just to the right of the tail and then ending at the neck. Repeat the process to the left of the tail. Remove the backbone and reserve for broth-making. With the chicken still breast-down in the sink, look for the sternum—a large piece of cartilage in the middle of the breast. Pierce or cut it with the shears. Now, flip the chicken over, flattening the breast.

4 Dry the chicken off thoroughly with paper towels and place it on top of the dish with the vegetables.

5 Combine the remaining 1 teaspoon sea salt, garlic powder, onion powder, and a pinch of cinnamon in a small bowl. Sprinkle over the chicken and rub to coat evenly. Make sure to cover every last bit!

6 Bake for 50 minutes, and then check for doneness with a thermometer—cook until the internal temperature measured at the thickest part of the breast is 165°F. Depending on the size of the bird, it could take 90 minutes or more to cook. If you notice the wings starting to burn, cover them with foil as the rest of the chicken continues to cook.

7 Serve warm with the pan juices.

STORAGE: Keeps in the refrigerator for about a week.

VARIATION: You can use turnips or parsnips, if you can't find rutabagas.

2	pounds rutabagas (about 2), chopped into 1-inch chunks
5	large carrots, chopped into 1-inch chunks
1	green apple, cored and chopped into 1-inch chunks
2	tablespoons solid cooking fat (page 170), melted
1½	tablespoons minced fresh thyme
½	teaspoon ground turmeric
1½	teaspoons sea salt, divided
	Ground cinnamon
1	pastured chicken (4–5 pounds)
½	teaspoon garlic powder
½	teaspoon onion powder

HERBED SEAFOOD BAKE
WITH BACON-RADICCHIO SALAD

TIME: 25 MINUTES
SERVES: 2

SEAFOOD

1	pound mussels, scrubbed (see Note)
1	pound littleneck clams, scrubbed (see Note)
½	pound raw jumbo shrimp, deveined
	Fresh thyme sprigs
	Fresh marjoram sprigs
	Fresh oregano sprigs
3	cloves garlic, minced
1	tablespoon sea salt
2	tablespoons olive oil
1	tablespoon chopped fresh parsley

SALAD

3	slices bacon, fried crisp and crumbled
1	pear, cored and chopped
1	small head radicchio, chopped
1	head endive, chopped
1	tablespoon olive oil
1	tablespoon white balsamic vinegar

1 Preheat the oven to 450°F. Line a large baking sheet with parchment paper.

2 Place the seafood on the baking sheet and top with the thyme, marjoram, and oregano sprigs, garlic, and sea salt. Place in the oven and roast for 15 minutes, or until most of the shells have opened. If any mussels or clams remain unopened, discard, as this may indicate they are bad.

3 While the seafood is roasting, combine all of the salad ingredients in a serving bowl and toss to combine.

4 You will know the seafood is finished cooking when the shrimp is pink and opaque. Remove from the oven, transfer to a serving dish, drizzle with olive oil, and sprinkle with parsley. Serve with the salad on the side.

STORAGE: Shellfish and salad don't keep well, so serve fresh.

NOTE: To clean shellfish, start by discarding any broken shells and rinsing under cold running water. Transfer to a large pot of cold salted water and refrigerate for 30 minutes. Instead of straining the shellfish, lift them individually out of the pot so that the sediment stays at the bottom. If there is any debris or are "beards" on the mussels, pinch them off before cooking.

VARIATION: This recipe can easily be doubled to serve 4 people. It is extremely easy, but looks elegant and sophisticated for a dinner party.

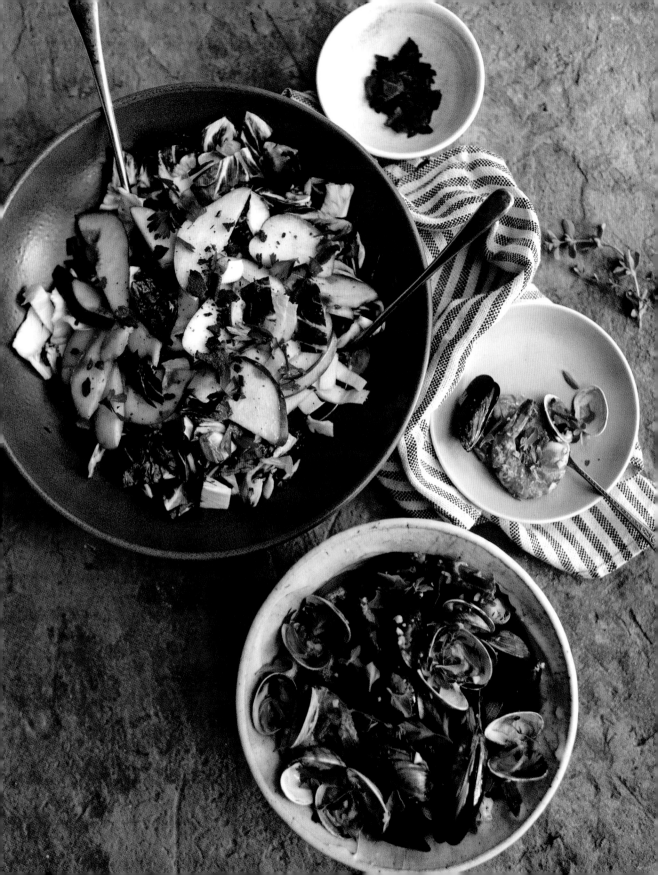

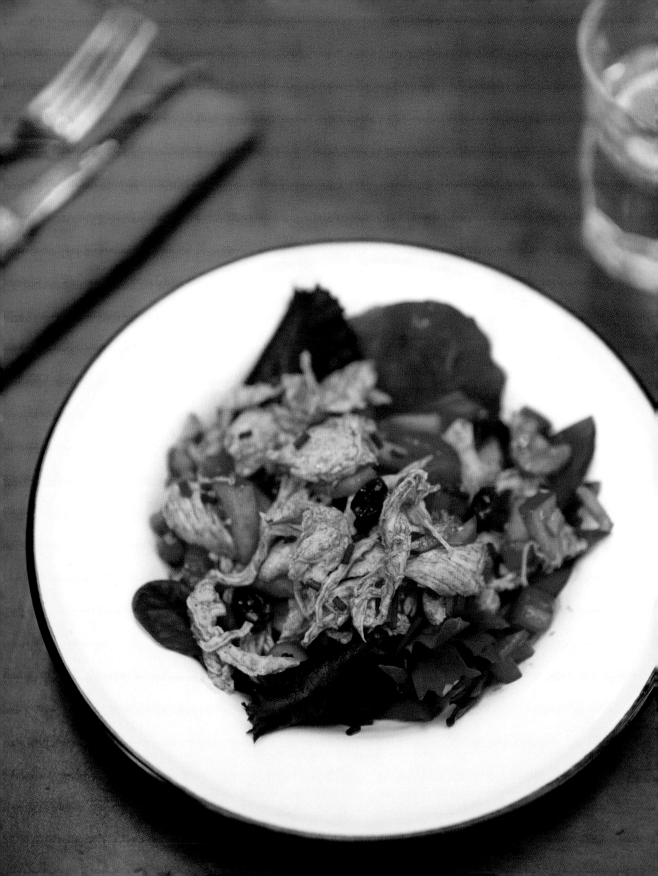

CURRIED CHICKEN SALAD

TIME: 45 MINUTES
SERVES: 4

1 Heat the solid cooking fat in a skillet over medium heat. When the fat has melted and the pan is hot, cook the chicken, top-side down, for 5 to 7 minutes, or until lightly browned.

2 Flip each piece of chicken, add the broth, cover, and lower the heat so that it simmers. Cook for 15 to 20 minutes, or until the internal temperature measured at the thickest part of the breast reaches 165°F.

3 Meanwhile, combine the celery, carrots, apples, onions, garlic, and currants or raisins in a large bowl and set aside.

4 Place all of the dressing ingredients in a small bowl and whisk until well combined. Add to the bowl with the vegetables, stir to combine, and set aside.

5 Remove the chicken from the pan and set aside to cool. Once it is cool enough to handle safely, or using two forks, shred the breast meat.

6 Add the chicken to the bowl with the vegetables and dressing, stir well to combine, and serve on a bed of salad greens, garnished with the chives.

STORAGE: Keeps for several days in the refrigerator.

SALAD

1	tablespoon solid cooking fat (page 170)
1½	pounds pastured chicken breasts
1	cup Bone Broth (page 168)
4	ribs celery, finely chopped
2	large carrots, finely chopped
1	green apple, cored and finely chopped
½	red onion, minced
2	cloves garlic, minced
½	cup currants or raisins
½	pound mixed salad greens, for serving
	Chives, finely chopped, for garnish

DRESSING

¾	cup olive oil
	Juice of 1 lemon
1	teaspoon apple cider vinegar
1	teaspoon ground turmeric
¾	teaspoon sea salt
½	teaspoon ground cinnamon

COLD "NOODLE" AND SALMON SALAD

TIME: 35 MINUTES
SERVES: 4

SALAD

1½	pounds wild-caught salmon, cut into 4 servings
	Sea salt, to taste
4	green onions, chopped
2	large zucchini
½	bunch radishes, ends removed and very thinly sliced (about 1½ cups)

DRESSING

2	cups chopped parsley
¾	cup olive oil
	Zest and juice of ½ lemon
2	teaspoons minced capers

1 Preheat the oven to 400°F.

2 Place the salmon, skin-side down, on a baking sheet and season with the sea salt. Top with the green onions. Bake for 15 minutes, depending on the thickness of the fillet. To tell if it is finished, its flesh should no longer be translucent, and it should flake with a fork.

3 While the salmon is baking, "spiralize" the zucchini using a spiralizer tool or a vegetable peeler to make long ribbons. Place in a large bowl, and add the radishes.

4 Place all of the dressing ingredients in a jar, close the lid tightly, and shake to combine. Pour the dressing over the zucchini salad, and toss to combine.

5 Serve the salad topped with the salmon.

STORAGE: Keeps for 2 to 3 days; store dressing separately.

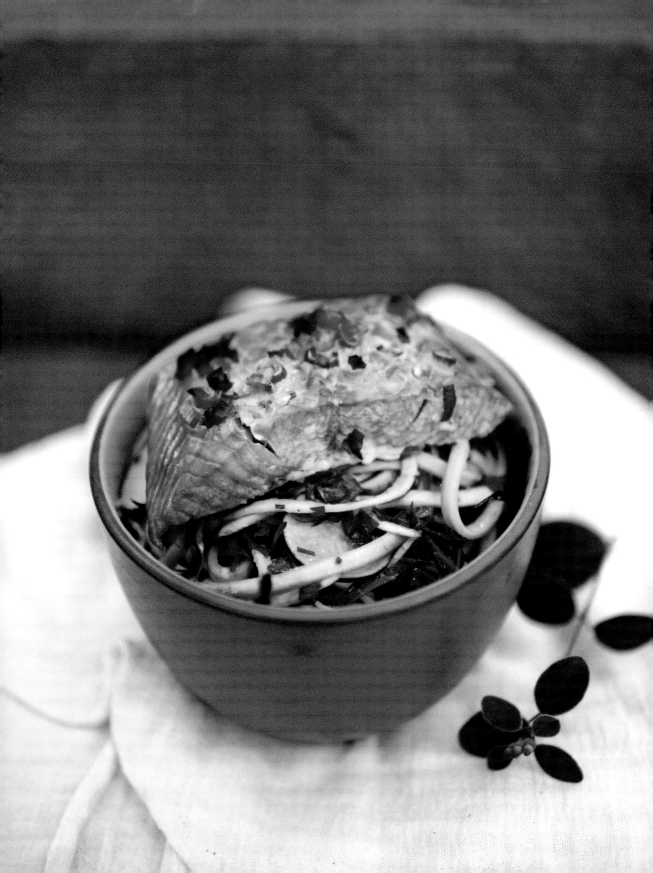

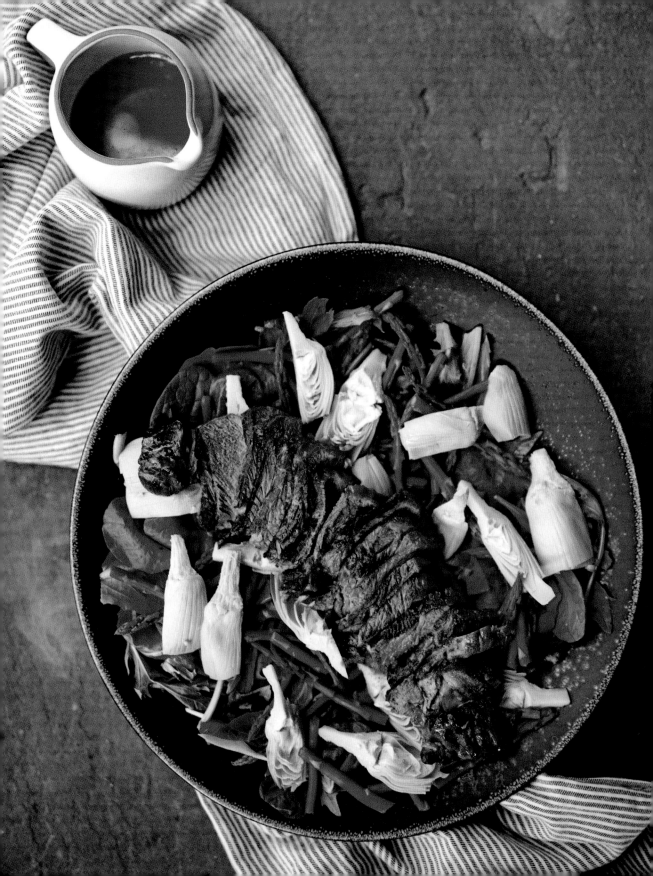

STEAK SALAD WITH SPRING VEGGIES

1 Place the asparagus in a pot and cover with water. Bring to a boil on high heat with the lid on. Immediately remove from heat, drain, and set aside.

2 Place all of the dressing ingredients into a jar, close the lid tightly, and shake to combine. Set aside.

3 Add the greens, artichokes, and asparagus to a large serving bowl and toss to combine.

4 Move the oven rack to the top and preheat the broiler. Rub the steak on both sides with salt, to taste.

5 Heat the solid cooking fat in the bottom of a cast-iron, ovenproof skillet on high heat. When the fat has melted and the pan is hot, sear the steak for 30 seconds on each side and carefully move the pan to the oven. Broil the steak for 2 minutes per side.

6 When the steak is finished, move it to a plate, loosely tent with foil, and allow to rest for 5 minutes. Slice the steak as thinly as possible.

7 Add the warm, thinly sliced steak and half of the dressing to the salad ingredients and toss to combine.

8 Serve with the remaining dressing or store it in an airtight jar in the refrigerator.

STORAGE: Keeps for 3 days in the refrigerator, dressing and salad stored separately.

TIME: 20 MINUTES
SERVES: 4

SALAD

1 bunch asparagus spears, woody ends removed, chopped in half

3 cups packed mixed greens

1 cup quartered artichoke hearts (canned, packed in water, and drained)

1 pound grass-fed beef steak (ribeye or New York strip works well)

   Sea salt

1 tablespoon solid cooking fat (page 170)

DRESSING

1/2 cup olive oil

2 tablespoons red wine vinegar

1 small shallot, minced

3 cloves garlic, minced

TUNA SALAD WITH AVO OR GARLIC "MAYO"

TIME: 20 MINUTES
SERVES: 3 OR 4

AVOCADO MAYO

1   avocado

$1/2$ cup olive oil

$1/4$ cup water

$1/2$ lemon, juiced

1   clove garlic

$1/2$ teaspoon turmeric

$1/2$ teaspoon sea salt

GARLIC MAYO

$1/2$ cup coconut concentrate, warmed (also known as coconut manna or coconut butter; see Note)

$1/2$ cup hot water

$1/4$ cup olive oil

3–4 cloves garlic

$1/4$ teaspoon sea salt

SALAD

1   (12-ounce) can tuna, drained

3   ribs celery, finely chopped

1   carrot, finely chopped

3   radishes, finely chopped

$1/2$ cup grapes, halved

1   tablespoon minced fresh dill

   Fresh salad greens

1 Place all of the mayo ingredients for the flavor you choose in a blender and blend on high for a minute or two, until a thick sauce forms (when freshly made, it should resemble the consistency of conventional mayo). If the sauce is too thick, thin with water until the desired consistency is reached.

2 Combine the tuna, celery, carrots, radishes, grapes, and dill in a bowl with the mayo and stir to combine.

3 Serve on top of a bed of fresh salad greens.

STORAGE: Keeps for a few days in the refrigerator. Garlic mayo will harden in the refrigerator but softens up after 20 minutes at room temperature.

NOTE: In order to measure the coconut concentrate, it is best to soften it in a warm-water bath before use, as it is solid at room temperature. For brand recommendations, see Resources on page 261.

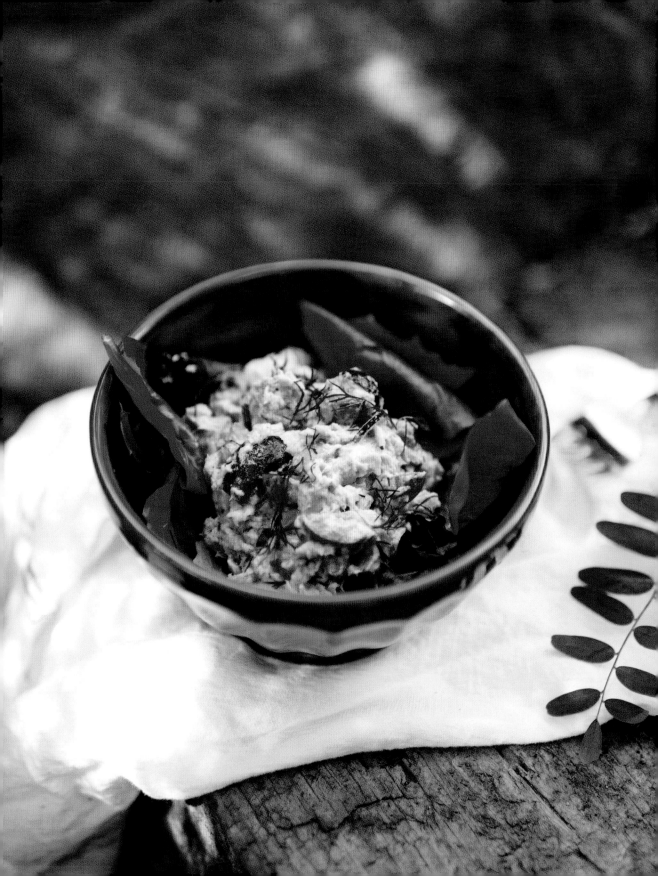

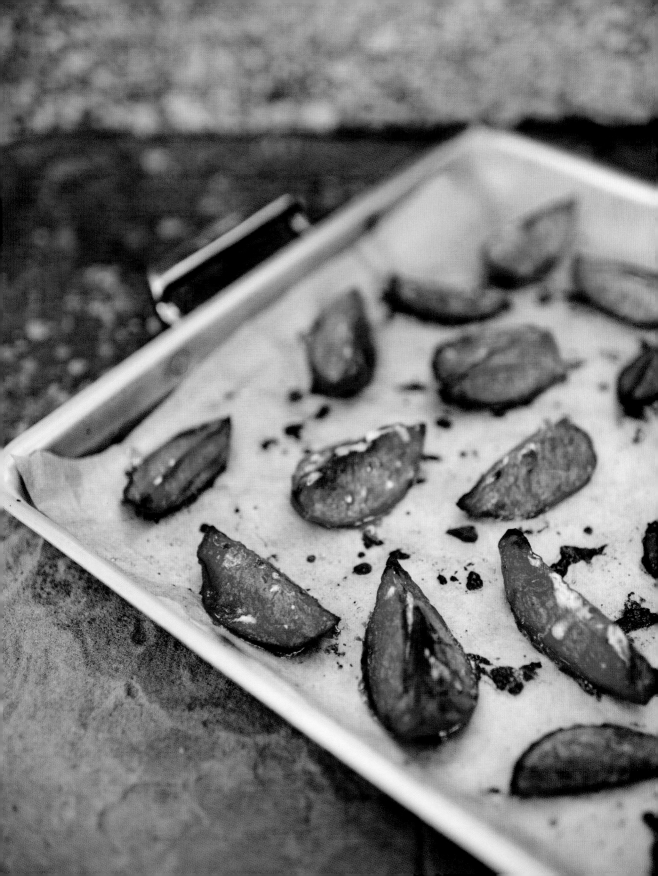

ROASTED STONE FRUIT

1 Preheat the oven to 425°F. Place the juice, coconut oil, ginger, cinnamon, and sea salt in a medium bowl and whisk to combine.

2 Add the fruit to the bowl and stir until evenly coated with the mixture. Place the pieces of fruit on a parchment paper–lined baking sheet, giving them plenty of space between, sprinkling with remaining liquid (if there is any!).

3 Cook for 20 minutes, or until the edges are browned and the fruit is soft. Serve warm.

STORAGE: Keeps for a few days in the refrigerator.

NOTE: If the fruit is more ripe than firm, it may take only 10 minutes to cook. Make sure to check in while cooking, if your fruit is already soft!

VARIATION: This recipe works well with other stone fruit, like apricots, as well as other types of fruit like apples and pears (although you will want to decrease the temperature to 375°F and increase the cooking time up to 20 additional minutes for these varieties).

TIME: 35 MINUTES
SERVES: 4

1/2	orange, juiced (about 2 tablespoons)
1	tablespoon coconut oil, melted
1/4	teaspoon ground ginger
1/4	teaspoon ground cinnamon
1/4	teaspoon sea salt
2	firm peaches, quartered and pits removed
2	firm nectarines, quartered and pits removed

LEMON PIE DATE BALLS

TIME: 15 MINUTES
MAKES: 8

Zest of 1 small lemon

¼ cup unsweetened coconut flakes

½ teaspoon sea salt

1 tablespoon lemon juice

2 cups dates, pitted

½ teaspoon ground ginger

1 whole vanilla bean, minced

2 tablespoons coconut concentrate (also known as coconut manna or coconut butter; see Note)

1 Combine the lemon zest, coconut flakes, and sea salt in a shallow bowl and set aside.

2 Combine the remaining ingredients in a food processor, and pulse to process until a "ball" forms. If the mixture is still too dry, add 1 teaspoon of water at a time until it does form a "ball."

3 Roll the mixture into approximately 8 small balls, and then roll through the lemon zest mixture to coat. Place on a parchment paper–lined plate, and transfer to the freezer for 5 minutes to harden.

STORAGE: Transfer to an airtight container for storage in the refrigerator. Keeps for a couple weeks; also freezes well.

NOTE: In order to measure the coconut concentrate, it is best to soften it in a warm-water bath before use, as it is solid at room temperature. For brand recommendations, see Resources on page 261. If you find yourself sensitive to vanilla bean seeds, scrape out the seeds and just use the pod.

The Autoimmune Wellness Handbook

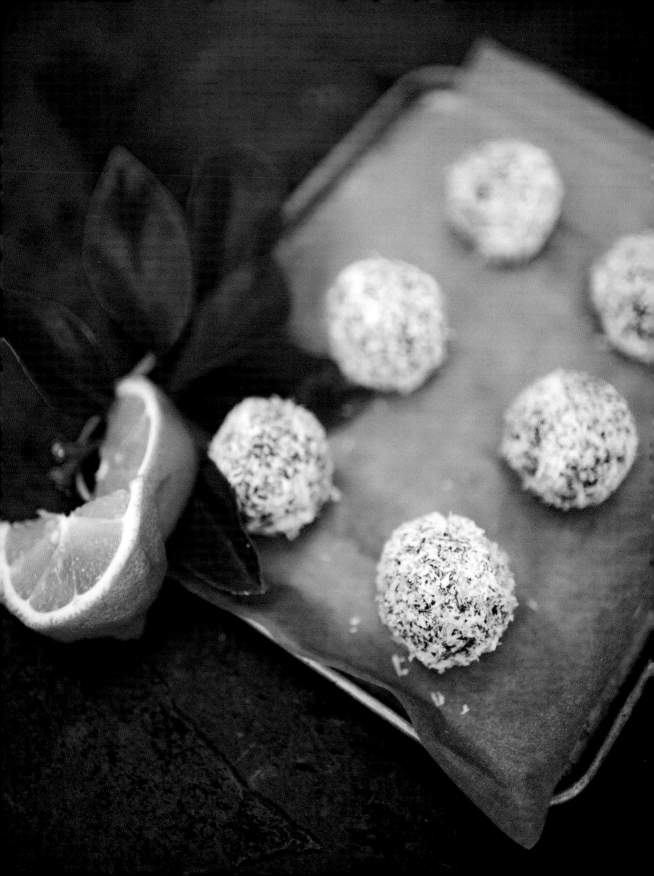

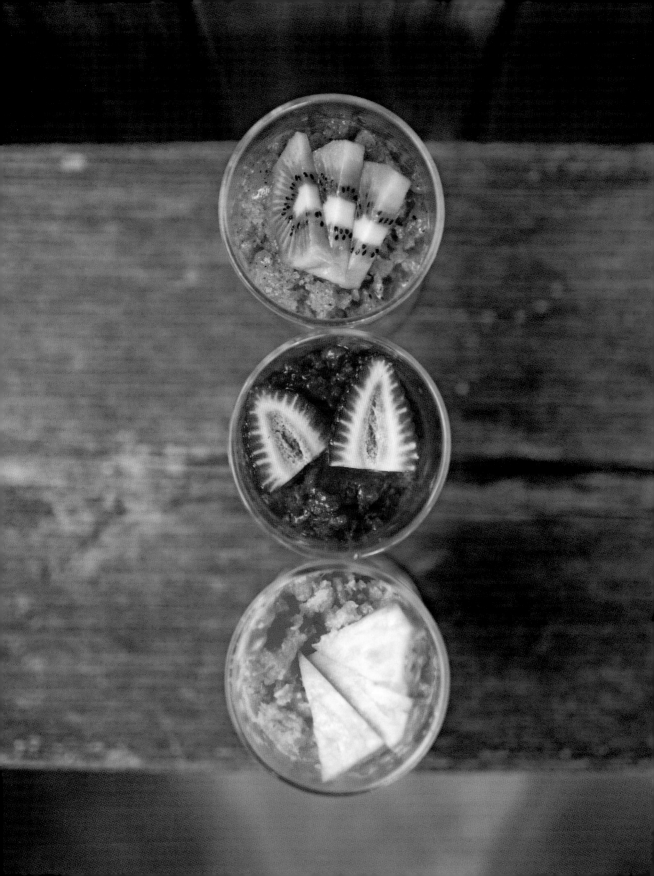

GRANITAS

1 Add all ingredients for the flavor you are making to a blender or food processor and process until smooth.

2 Pour into a 9 by 13-inch baking dish and place in the freezer, being sure to rake with the tines of a fork every 30 minutes for 4 hours, or until a "slushy" consistency develops.

STORAGE: Freezes well for several weeks.

NOTE: To make simple syrup, in a small saucepan, bring 1 cup honey and 1 cup water to a boil; simmer until the honey completely dissolves, about 3 minutes. Remove from the heat and let cool completely. Syrup stores in a glass jar for up to 1 month in the refrigerator.

TIME: 15 MINUTES, PLUS 4 HOURS TO CHILL
SERVES: 4

KIWI-LIME
- 4 kiwifruits, peeled and chopped
- Juice of 1 lime
- ¼ cup simple syrup (see **Note**)
- ¼ cup unflavored coconut water

STRAWBERRY "MARGARITA"
- 2 cups hulled and chopped strawberries
- Juice of 1 lime
- ¼ cup simple syrup (see **Note**)
- ¼ cup unflavored coconut water

PIÑA COLADA
- 2 cups chopped pineapple
- Juice of 1 lime
- ½ cup unflavored coconut water

RASPBERRY PUDDING

TIME: 15 MINUTES
SERVES: 4

3 ripe avocados

1³/₄ cups frozen raspberries

¹/₄ cup raw honey

3 tablespoons orange juice

¹/₂ vanilla bean, minced (see Note)

¹/₄ teaspoon sea salt

Raspberries, for garnish

Mint leaves, for garnish

1 Place all ingredients in a food processor or a high-powered blender and mix until thoroughly combined, about 30 seconds, stopping to scrape down the sides, if needed.

2 Serve garnished with raspberries and mint leaves.

STORAGE: Keeps in the refrigerator for a few days, but loses its color. Freezes well.

NOTE: If you find yourself sensitive to vanilla bean seeds, scrape out the seeds and just use the pod.

VARIATION: You can substitute other berries for this recipe—strawberries and blackberries both work well.

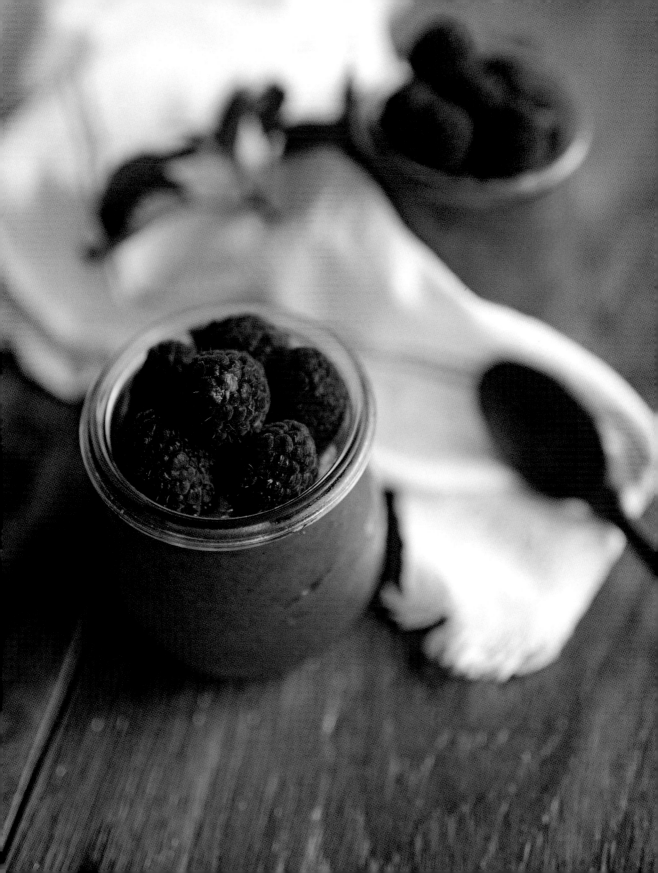

NO-BAKE LEMON-VANILLA "CHEESECAKE"

TIME: 1 HOUR, PLUS 24 HOURS TO SET
SERVES: 8

CRUST

1½	cups dried figs (about 7 ounces)
½	cup dried dates (about 2½ ounces)
½	cup unsweetened coconut flakes
1	tablespoon arrowroot starch
1	tablespoon melted coconut oil + additional for greasing the pan
	Pinch of sea salt

FILLING

1	cup filtered water
2	teaspoons grass-fed gelatin
1	cup coconut concentrate, melted (also known as coconut manna or coconut butter; see Notes)
½	cup raw honey, melted
½	cup lemon juice (from about 4 lemons)
2	tablespoons lemon zest (from about 2 lemons)
1	whole vanilla bean, minced (see Notes)
¼	teaspoon sea salt
	Fresh figs, for garnish
	Mint sprigs, for garnish

1 Place the dried figs, dates, coconut flakes, arrowroot, 1 tablespoon coconut oil, and sea salt in a food processor and process on high until a thick, sticky, homogenous paste forms (30 to 45 seconds). Grease an 8" springform cake pan with additional coconut oil, add the crust mixture, and spread evenly into the bottom of the pan with your fingers. Put it in the refrigerator to cool while you make the filling.

2 Place the water in a small saucepan and sprinkle the gelatin on top, giving it a few minutes to absorb some of the liquid and "bloom."

3 Meanwhile, combine the coconut concentrate, honey, lemon juice, lemon zest, vanilla bean, and sea salt in a blender or a food processor and blend on high for 30 seconds to combine. Set aside.

4 Place the saucepan with the gelatin on the stove and turn the heat on low. Heat the mixture very gently, stirring, only about 30 seconds or until the gelatin has dissolved completely. Do not let it get more than lukewarm.

5 Add the gelatin mixture to the blender or food processor with the rest of the filling ingredients and blend again, on high, until everything is well incorporated.

6 Pour onto the crust and cool in the refrigerator until firm, about 24 hours.

7 Garnish with fresh figs and mint, if desired.

STORAGE: Keeps for a week in the refrigerator. Keep cool for best texture. Do not freeze.

NOTES: In order to measure the coconut concentrate, it is best to soften it in a warm-water bath before use, as it is solid at room temperature. For brand recommendations, see Resources on page 261. If you find yourself sensitive to vanilla bean seeds, scrape out the seeds and just use the pod.

VARIATION: If fresh figs aren't in season, feel free to make this cake any time of year using other fresh fruit as a garnish. Berries or stone fruit would be great options.

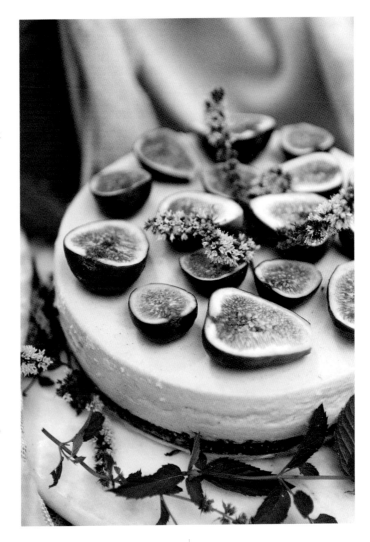

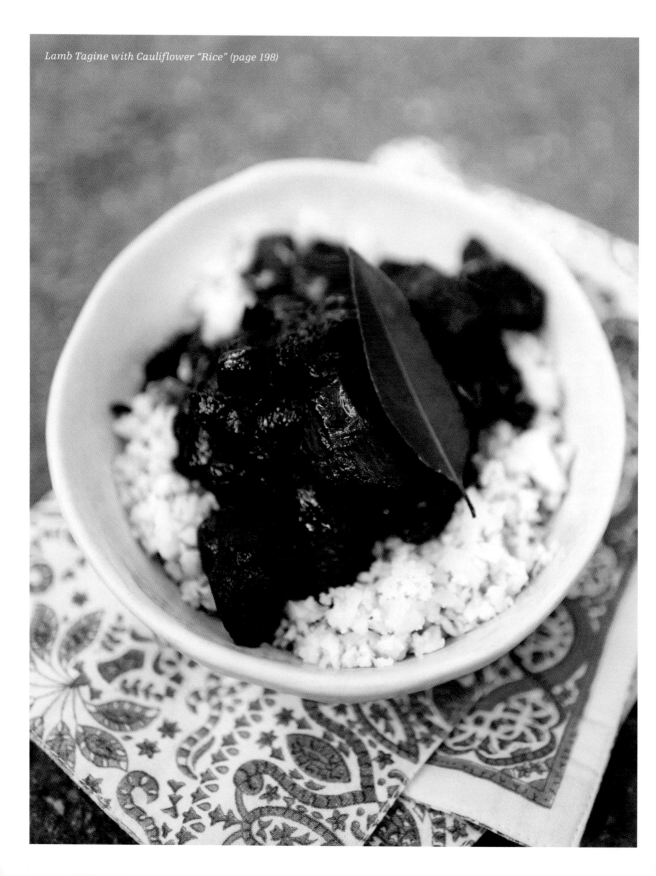

Lamb Tagine with Cauliflower "Rice" (page 198)

4-Week Meal Plan

INTRODUCTION

If you'd like to give the Autoimmune Protocol a try, it is best to *set yourself up for success*. What does that mean? The difference between making it happen and succumbing to temptation only a few days in is a good measure of planning and preparation. If you've done the work to make sure your kitchen is free of all of the inflammatory foods you no longer want to be eating and have replaced them with healing, nutrient-dense meals, there will be less chance of straying in weaker moments. Trust us—having been there, planning is the key to success in making these long-term dietary changes stick. Plus, once you start feeling better, it will be more motivation to continue!

The two big secrets to being prepared for the elimination phase are meal planning and batch-cooking. Meal planning is the practice of mapping out your meals for the week and letting that guide your shopping list and cooking days. Batch-cooking is the practice of cooking large batches of recipes to be enjoyed later, as a way to maximize time spent in the kitchen. Nobody wants to feel like a short-order cook, preparing three meals a day from scratch, especially when other family members are involved! Using the magical combination of meal planning and batch-cooking, you can reduce your time in the kitchen to four or five sessions per week, while still providing yourself all of the food you need for *every* meal.

In order to take all of the planning and guesswork out of figuring out what to eat, we have included a 4-week meal plan along with all of the supplemental resources you need to get started—pantry basics, shopping lists, a food selection guide, and a tool list. Make sure to read all of the accompanying material in this chapter, as it includes important information for personalizing and making the most of your protocol.

Notes about the Meal Plan and Shopping List

- All of the recipes included in the meal plan are suitable for the elimination phase of the Autoimmune Protocol—no grains, beans, legumes, dairy, eggs, nuts, seeds, or nightshade vegetables or spices.

- The meal plan feeds 1 person for 4 weeks, accounting for generous servings of food at mealtimes and to eat as snacks. In the beginning, it is important to make sure to have an abundance of food to avoid a situation where you are hungry and there is nothing to eat! If you find that the quantity is too much, you can easily freeze some servings of soups or stews to eat later (and then just think—you will be that much further ahead!).

- We have accounted for 4 to 6 ounces of meat per meal in the shopping lists and recipes. If you want to eat more or less, you can tweak this level accordingly. None of the recipes is so specific that a slight change in meat quantity will make a difference.

- If you will be feeding more than just yourself, you will need to make adjustments to the meal plan (like adding some portions or sides to the meals).

- The twice-weekly shopping lists include all of the food called for on the meal plan (not including optional snacks) and assume that you will be cooking midday (lunch) on Sundays and end-of-day (dinner) on Wednesdays.

Time Management

- Meals that need to be cooked from scratch are noted in bold type and those in regular type have already been prepped and cooked and only need a quick reheat or assembly. You can easily glance at the week and see which mealtimes will require more time for preparation. You can expect to do more cooking in the evenings and on weekends and little cooking from scratch at breakfast or lunch.

- Note that a couple of times a week, there are indications to thaw portions of previously frozen meals for the following day, or cook meals for the following day. For the latter, you can choose to cook these breakfasts fresh in the morning, or prep them the night before if you lack time early in the day.

- Plan on spending some time batch-cooking on the weekend for the upcoming week. If you don't work a traditional workweek, shift the days so that the big cooking days fall when you have more time.

- If you are rendering your own solid cooking fat (page 170) and/or making your own Bone Broth (page 168), schedule a time to do this before you embark on the meal plan so you have those ingredients ready. They will be called for in the recipes, so plan ahead!

- You will need to budget enough time to make two trips to the grocery store during the week. If you would like to gather everything in one trip that is fine, just take into account how long the meat will last in the refrigerator and set a freezing and thawing schedule if it is going to be too long before cooking.

Storing and Reheating Food

- Before you begin batch-cooking, make sure that you have enough storage containers. See the Tool List section on page 236 for more details.

- To reheat meals, you can use a skillet, pot, oven, or microwave, whatever is your preference. Our favorite way is to use an oven-safe glass container in a low (300°F) oven for 20 minutes.

- For the meals that are to be frozen, if you are using glass, make sure to use no larger than a wide-mouth pint jar filled appropriately to the freeze line. Any jar with shoulders, or larger than this, is likely to crack.

- To thaw frozen meals, place the container in a warm-water bath for a couple of hours or directly in the refrigerator for 24 hours.

Other Notes

- Pay attention to the pantry items section on the shopping list and make sure that you are keeping them in stock—things like garlic, spices, cooking fats, and so on. The recipes in the meal plan will call on those items frequently, and they won't be included on the regular shopping list.

- Pay attention to the tool list and make sure you have all of the items

required. We don't call for any unusual or expensive equipment, but there are a few common tools you will want to make sure you have in your kitchen, as well as containers to store your meals in once they are cooked.

- If you have any sensitivities or food preferences beyond what is omitted in the elimination phase, the meal plan can serve as a framework for you to customize. Many of the recipes come with substitution ideas.

Snacks and Treats

- You'll notice the meal plan does not include recipes for snacks. Snacks tend to be highly individual, with some people needing them and others fine with three generous meals. In order to minimize waste and to make the meal plan fit more people's needs, we have left you with generous portions that can be eaten as snacks, or you can freeze the leftovers and have some elimination phase–friendly snacks around, like fruit.

- Treats are best left for special occasions. Too much sugar can seriously undermine healing. If you can't live without a treat, you can make one of the treat recipes earlier in this chapter (pages 215 to 223), but try to limit it to once or twice a month, especially when you first begin.

Autoimmune Wellness Handbook
4-Week Meal Plan

	BREAKFAST	LUNCH	DINNER	ALSO PREP
WEEK 1				
PREP DAY		Green Breakfast Soup (page 180)	Tuna Salad with Avo or Garlic "Mayo" (page 212)	Bone Broth (page 168) (freeze all but 3 cups)
MONDAY	Green Breakfast Soup	Tuna Salad	Beef Curry Soup (page 193)	
TUESDAY	Green Breakfast Soup	Tuna Salad	Beef Curry Soup	Freeze 3 servings Green Breakfast Soup
WEDNESDAY	Green Breakfast Soup	Tuna Salad	Beef Curry Soup	Butternut Breakfast Bake (page 177)
THURSDAY	Butternut Breakfast Bake	Beef Curry Soup	Lamb Tagine with Cauliflower "Rice" (page 198)	
FRIDAY	Butternut Breakfast Bake	Lamb Tagine	Spatchcocked Chicken with Tumeric Veggies (page 203)	
SATURDAY	Butternut Breakfast Bake	Lamb Tagine	Spatchcocked Chicken	
SUNDAY	Butternut Breakfast Bake	Spatchcocked Chicken	Emerald Salmon with Zesty Green Sauce (page 199)	Double Pork Pesto Patties with Wilted Chard (page 182)

Autoimmune Wellness Handbook
4-Week Meal Plan

	BREAKFAST	LUNCH	DINNER	ALSO PREP
WEEK 2				
MONDAY	Double Pork Pesto Patties	Spatchcocked Chicken	Emerald Salmon	Thaw 2 cups Bone Broth (page 168)
TUESDAY	Double Pork Pesto Patties	Emerald Salmon	**Hidden Liver Chili (page 189)**	
WEDNESDAY	Double Pork Pesto Patties	Hidden Liver Chili	**Curried Chicken Salad (page 207)**	
THURSDAY	Double Pork Pesto Patties	Curried Chicken Salad	Hidden Liver Chili	Thaw 3 servings Green Breakfast Soup
FRIDAY	Green Breakfast Soup	Curried Chicken Salad	Hidden Liver Chili	
SATURDAY	Green Breakfast Soup	Hidden Liver Chili	**Citrus-Ginger Brined Pork Roast (page 200)**	Thaw 1 cup Bone Broth
SUNDAY	Green Breakfast Soup	**Moroccan Chicken Thighs with Apricots and Olives (page 194)**	Citrus-Ginger Brined Pork Roast	**Nutrivore's Breakfast (page 178)** **Bone Broth (if needed)**

(continued)

Autoimmune Wellness Handbook
4-Week Meal Plan

	BREAKFAST	LUNCH	DINNER	ALSO PREP
WEEK 3				
MONDAY	Nutrivore's Breakfast	Moroccan Chicken Thighs	Citrus-Ginger Brined Pork Roast	
TUESDAY	Nutrivore's Breakfast	Moroccan Chicken Thighs	Citrus-Ginger Brined Pork Roast	Thaw 2 cups Bone Broth
WEDNESDAY	Nutrivore's Breakfast	Moroccan Chicken Thighs	**Balsamic Beef Stew (page 185)**	
THURSDAY	Nutrivore's Breakfast	Balsamic Beef Stew	**Lemongrass-Scented Chicken Stew (page 190)**	
FRIDAY	Nutrivore's Breakfast	Lemongrass-Scented Chicken Stew	Balsamic Beef Stew	Freeze 3 servings Lemongrass-Scented Chicken Stew
SATURDAY	Nutrivore's Breakfast	Lemongrass-Scented Chicken Stew	Balsamic Beef Stew	
SUNDAY	**Green Breakfast Soup (page 180)**	**Emerald Salmon with Zesty Green Sauce (page 199)**	**Apple-Beet Burgers with Parsnip Fries and Horseradish Spread (page 197)**	**Bone Broth** (if needed)

Autoimmune Wellness Handbook
4-Week Meal Plan

	BREAKFAST	LUNCH	DINNER	ALSO PREP
WEEK 4				
MONDAY	Green Breakfast Soup	Emerald Salmon	Apple-Beet Burgers	Freeze 3 cups Green Breakfast Soup
TUESDAY	Green Breakfast Soup	Emerald Salmon	Apple-Beet Burgers	**Pork Patties (page 182) Thaw 3 servings of chicken stew**
WEDNESDAY	Double Pork Pesto Patties	Apple-Beet Burgers	Lemongrass-Scented Chicken Stew	Thaw 2 cups Bone Broth
THURSDAY	Double Pork Pesto Patties	Lemongrass-Scented Chicken Stew	**Beef Curry Soup (page 193)**	
FRIDAY	Double Pork Pesto Patties	Lemongrass-Scented Chicken Stew	Beef Curry Soup	
SATURDAY	Double Pork Pesto Patties	**Tuna Salad with Avo or Garlic "Mayo" (page 212)**	Beef Curry Soup	Thaw 1 serving Green Breakfast Soup
SUNDAY	Green Breakfast Soup	Tuna Salad	Beef Curry Soup	

Week 1
Shopping List

PANTRY ITEMS	SUNDAY	WEDNESDAY
Solid cooking fat of your choice (lard, tallow, duck fat, etc.; see page 170)	1 large, whole pastured chicken (5–6 pounds)	1½ pounds grass-fed ground beef
Coconut oil	2 pounds bones (see page 168)	1 (4–5 pounds) pasture-raised chicken
Extra-virgin olive oil	1½ pounds grass-fed beef stew meat	1 pound lamb stew meat
Full-fat coconut milk (BPA- and thickener-free)	1 (12-ounce) can tuna, packed in water	1 butternut squash
Raw honey	2 large sweet potatoes	2 rutabagas (or 4 parsnips)
Apple cider vinegar	4 large parsnips	1 pound carrots
Balsamic vinegar	1 pound carrots	1 small red onion
Onion powder	1 bunch celery	1 head cauliflower
Garlic powder	2 large zucchini	3 leeks
Bay leaves	1 bunch Swiss chard	1 bunch fresh parsley
Sea salt	1 bunch kale	2 sweet apples
Ground turmeric	1 bunch radishes	1 green apple
Ground cinnamon	6 ounces fresh salad greens	½ cup dried apricots
Ground cloves	2 cups button mushrooms	½ cup prunes
Ground ginger	1 avocado or coconut concentrate*	1½ cups raisins
Yellow onions	1 bunch cilantro	Fresh thyme
Fresh garlic	Fresh dill	1 lemon
Fresh ginger	1 bunch green onions	
	1 lime	
	2 lemons	
	½ cup grapes	

*depending on the recipe variation you choose

The Autoimmune Wellness Handbook

Week 2
Shopping List

PANTRY ITEMS	SUNDAY	WEDNESDAY
Solid cooking fat of your choice (lard, tallow, duck fat, etc.; see page 170)	2 pounds grass-fed ground beef	2–3 pounds pastured pork roast
Coconut oil	1 pound pastured ground pork	2 pounds boneless, skin-on chicken thighs
Extra-virgin olive oil	1 pound wild-caught salmon fillet	$1\frac{1}{2}$ pounds pastured chicken breast
Full-fat coconut milk (BPA- and thickener-free)	$\frac{1}{2}$ pound grass-fed beef liver	1 pound carrots (if needed)
Raw honey	1 pound bacon	1 bunch celery (if needed)
Apple cider vinegar	3 parsnips	1 red onion (if needed)
Balsamic vinegar	1 pound carrots	6 ounces fresh salad greens
Onion powder	1 crown broccoli	$\frac{1}{2}$ cup green olives (without pimento)
Garlic powder	1 bunch asparagus	Fresh thyme (if needed)
Bay leaves	1 bulb fennel	Fresh oregano (if needed)
Sea salt	2 large bunches rainbow chard	$\frac{1}{2}$ cup dried apricots
Ground turmeric	1 bunch celery (if needed)	$\frac{1}{2}$ cup currants or raisins
Ground cinnamon	1 bunch cilantro	6 oranges (or 1 orange and $1\frac{1}{2}$ cups orange juice)
Ground cloves	Fresh basil	1 green apple
Ground ginger	Fresh oregano	2 lemons
Yellow onions	1 avocado	
Fresh garlic	2 lemons	
Fresh ginger		

Week 3
Shopping List

PANTRY ITEMS	SUNDAY	WEDNESDAY
Solid cooking fat of your choice (lard, tallow, duck fat, etc.; see page 170)	2 pounds grass-fed ground beef	2 (4–5 pounds) pasture-raised chickens
Coconut oil	$1\frac{1}{2}$ pounds grass-fed beef stew meat	2 large sweet potatoes
Extra-virgin olive oil	$\frac{1}{4}$ pound grass-fed beef liver	1 large butternut squash
Full-fat coconut milk (BPA- and thickener-free)	2 pounds bones (if needed)	2 large zucchini
Raw honey	4 large sweet potatoes	2 cups button mushrooms
Apple cider vinegar	2 pounds carrots	1 bunch Swiss chard
Balsamic vinegar	1 bunch celery (if needed)	1 bunch green onions
Onion powder	1 bunch kale	4 stalks lemongrass
Garlic powder	Fresh rosemary	Fresh turmeric (use ground if you can't find fresh)
Bay leaves	Fresh oregano (if needed)	1 bunch cilantro
Sea salt	Fresh thyme (if needed)	1 avocado
Ground turmeric		2 lemons
Ground cinnamon		
Ground cloves		
Ground ginger		
Yellow onions		
Fresh garlic		
Fresh ginger		

The Autoimmune Wellness Handbook

Week 4
Shopping List

PANTRY ITEMS	SUNDAY	WEDNESDAY
Solid cooking fat of your choice (lard, tallow, duck fat, etc.; see page 170)	1 pound grass-fed ground beef	$1\frac{1}{2}$ pounds grass-fed beef stew meat
Coconut oil	1 pound pastured ground pork	1 (12-ounce) can tuna, packed in water
Extra-virgin olive oil	1 pound wild-caught salmon fillet	4 large parsnips
Full-fat coconut milk (BPA- and thickener-free)	$\frac{1}{2}$ pound bacon	1 pound carrots
Raw honey	2 pounds parsnips	1 bunch celery (if needed)
Apple cider vinegar	1 beet	1 bunch radishes
Balsamic vinegar	1 crown broccoli	1 bunch kale
Onion powder	1 bunch asparagus	6 ounces fresh salad greens
Garlic powder	1 bulb fennel	1 bunch cilantro
Bay leaves	$\frac{1}{2}$ pound fresh horseradish	Fresh dill
Sea salt	2 large bunches rainbow chard	1 avocado or coconut concentrate*
Ground turmeric	1 bunch cilantro	1 lime
Ground cinnamon	Fresh thyme (if needed)	1 lemon
Ground cloves	Fresh chives	$\frac{1}{2}$ cup grapes
Ground ginger	Fresh basil	
Yellow onions	1 apple	
Fresh garlic	1 lemon	
Fresh ginger		

*depending on the recipe variation you choose

TOOL LIST

Here is a list of all of the kitchen tools you will need to have handy in order to follow the 4-Week Meal Plan. None is out of the ordinary, but it is important to make sure that you have everything you need before you get started. We've also included a list of optional tools that make some tasks (like making broth) easier, but aren't required.

- Cutting board
- Sharp knife
- Large stockpot
- Skillet
- Large roasting dish
- Baking sheet
- Mixing bowls
- Blender
- Colander
- Glass containers for food storage
- Parchment paper
- Assorted mixing spoons
- Ladle
- Spatula
- Timer
- Measuring spoons/cups
- Pot holder
- Kitchen towels
- Pressure cooker or slow-cooker
- Box grater

Optional

- High-powered blender
- Food processor
- Pressure cooker or slow-cooker (as an additional tool)

- Extra stockpot
- Wide-mouth pint jars for freezing food

PANTRY GUIDE

In order to get your kitchen ready for the elimination phase, we recommend following our three-step pantry prep method for weeding out all of the foods that are likely temptations, as well as replacing those foods with nutritious alternatives.

Step #1: Get rid of all of the "bad stuff."

The first thing you should do is box up all of the foods you are unlikely to be eating again anytime soon—things like breads, pastas, flour, sugar, refined vegetable and seed oils, and anything processed that includes food chemicals and long ingredient lists. Donate it to the food pantry, and get it out of the house as soon as possible.

Step #2: Store all of the "maybe stuff."

There are likely foods lurking in your pantry that will be off-limits during the elimination phase, but you may be able to reintroduce them with success later. Instead of preemptively tossing these ingredients, we suggest packing them up in a box and placing them in a closet or somewhere inconvenient, to minimize temptation. This would include things like gluten-free products containing nuts and seeds (like spices, nut butters, or just the raw nuts and seeds themselves), nightshades, coffee, and chocolate. No need to give away or toss if you might be able to have them again in the future!

We highly recommend actually getting these items out of sight instead of letting them sit in your cabinets while you undertake your elimination phase. Put them in a box, tape it up, and bury it in a closet somewhere. There is nothing worse than the unnecessary temptation of that chocolate bar sitting in your cupboard begging to be eaten!

Step #3: Stock your pantry with Autoimmune Protocol–friendly ingredients.

With all that room you just made, invest in some ingredients you will be using for cooking elimination phase–friendly meals. While you don't need to go out and purchase everything on this list, at a minimum you will want some cooking fats, vinegar, some herbs and spices, and some baking ingredients should you decide to incorporate baking into your routine. Note that we don't call for many of these baking ingredients in the recipes in this book, but you may want to use them for experimenting or following other elimination-phase treat recipes you find.

The truth is, setting up your pantry for the Autoimmune Protocol is pretty simple, and you don't have to track down a bunch of exotic ingredients to make eating this way work. We suggest focusing mostly on finding a variety of high-quality cooking fats and spices to work with, rather than getting hung up on alternative flours, sweeteners, and snacks (which can be quite expensive!).

We've prioritized this list with the ingredients per category we think are most common in elimination phase–friendly recipes, with some mention of additional ingredients you may want to consider. For product recommendations for some of these ingredients, see Resources on page 261.

Alternative Flours

- **ARROWROOT STARCH/FLOUR**—This starch works well for thickening sauces or gravies, as well as baking. Most people are familiar with the small jars of it in the spice section, but it is available for a much better price in a bulk, bagged form.

- **CASSAVA FLOUR**—This flour is a newcomer on the scene and seems to create great texture when used in place of regular flour.

- **COCONUT FLOUR**—This is a common replacement in allergen-free baking that can be dry and difficult to work with. Most recipes use a blend of this flour with a starch like arrowroot or tapioca, which gives it a better consistency. Caution should be used for those who have a coconut sensitivity or don't do well with inulin fiber.

- **TAPIOCA STARCH/FLOUR**—This starch is similar to arrowroot and often interchangeable. Like arrowroot, it can be used to thicken, as well as for baking.

- Less common flours include plantain flour, tigernut flour, and sweet potato flour.

Sweeteners

- **COCONUT SUGAR**—This is a nice option when granulated sugar is called for, instead of a liquid one, in a recipe.

- **HONEY**—Raw, unpasteurized honey is nice to have on hand to sweeten tea and make occasional treats. Be cautious; different types of honey can have different textures, greatly affecting the outcome baked goods.

- **MAPLE SYRUP**—The delicious flavor maple brings is undeniable, and having some grade B in the pantry for treat-making can be handy.

- Less common sweeteners include coconut syrup, maple sugar, and dried fruit (like dates, raisins, etc.).

Coconut Products

- **COCONUT FLAKES**—Large-flake coconut is nice to eat as a snack (it's delicious toasted!) and the small-flake coconut can be used to make homemade coconut milk, as well as baked goods.

- **COCONUT MILK**—If you don't have a high-powered blender to make it at home, thickener-free coconut milk packed in BPA-free cans is a nice option to have for using in sauces, smoothies, and curries. (BPA is an endocrine-disrupting chemical.)

- **COCONUT WATER**—While probably too sweet to drink regularly, it is nice to have on hand as a rehydration beverage should someone in the family come down with a stomach bug. It is also used in the Granitas recipe on page 219.

- **COCONUT WRAPS**—These are a fun option for a quick meal; just wrap and go!

Cooking Fats

- **AVOCADO OIL**—This is a nice alternative to olive oil, and the same quality and bottle requirements apply because it also easily oxidizes.

- **COCONUT OIL**—A great, neutral-flavored fat that is nice to use for cooking and can be used as the solid cooking fat called for in our recipes, should you not have high-quality animal fats to render yourself.

- **EXTRA-VIRGIN OLIVE OIL**—Try to find a high-quality, cold-pressed, organic oil that is stored in an opaque bottle.

- **RENDERED SOLID COOKING FAT**—This is one ingredient you can't go without, as you will need it for cooking. Make your own using the recipe on page 170! Lard, tallow, and duck fat all work well here—if you can't make your own, check out Resources on page 261 for sourcing options.

- Less common cooking fats include palm shortening and red palm oil (choose sustainably harvested).

Preserved Meat

- **BEEF JERKY**—Make your own or buy a brand that does not contain nightshades, soy, or gluten.

- **CANNED FISH**—Buy tuna, salmon, sardines, or oysters, packed in extra-virgin olive oil or water and not in BPA-lined cans. Make sure that they do not contain off-limit spices or soybean oil!

- **EPIC BARS**—These are great pemmican (fat and protein) bars that have a much softer texture than jerky and make a great snack.

- **GELATIN**—This is a nice ingredient to use as a gut-healing supplement (a lot of folks will stir it into tea) or to texturize allergen-free desserts (such as No-Bake Lemon-Vanilla "Cheesecake" on page 222).

Assorted Foods and Flavorings

● **OLIVES**—If you can find them cured with salt only and not citric acid (derived from corn), these make an excellent snack. Beware of pimentos or other nightshade ingredients!

● **FISH SAUCE**—Use this to add umami to dishes (caution to those with histamine intolerance!).

● **COCONUT AMINOS**—This is a coconut-based soy sauce replacement that you can use in a stir-fry.

● **APPLE CIDER VINEGAR**—We recommend having at least one vinegar on hand to add to your meals, and this is an all-around standout that complements many flavors.

● Other flavorings include balsamic vinegar, white wine vinegar, red wine vinegar, and cooking wine.

Spices

● **DRIED HERBS**—Thyme, rosemary, dill, oregano, marjoram, and sage should get you started. Dried herbs aren't nearly as tasty as fresh, but they work great in a pinch.

● **GROUND SPICES**—Turmeric, ginger, garlic, cinnamon, and onion are a great start here. You can use these to make your own elimination phase–friendly curry blend instead of using the usual nightshade and seed spice version.

● **SALT**—It is nice to have a few different types of salt on hand. A good all-around sea salt is a must in any kitchen. Try some fun options like truffle sea salt and smoked sea salt to add some additional flavor.

● **SEAWEED**—There are many types of seaweeds you can use to make elimination phase–friendly sushi (like nori), or just a blend of flakes to sprinkle on top of dishes. This is a great way to add flavor and nutrients to your meals.

● **CAROB POWDER**—You can use this ingredient to make chocolate-like treats.

Snacks

● **SWEET POTATO CHIPS**—Look for a brand that is cooked in coconut oil instead of seed oils. These are great for plane travel or road trips!

● **PLANTAIN CHIPS**—You can find these in both sweet and savory varieties (using either ripe or green plantains).

● **SEAWEED SNACKS**—These are fun for when you are on the go!

SELECTING FOODS

There is no question that higher-quality foods confer greater health benefits. The way livestock is raised or produce is grown *does* affect its nutrient value. Those nutrients are the focus of the Autoimmune Protocol and are exactly what a body healing from autoimmune disease requires. That said, we are well aware that these foods are often high-priced and, in many cases, not all that easy to track down. Wouldn't it be amazing if every budget were big enough and every kitchen was within a few miles of an organic farm? Alas, we know that isn't reality! Before we start exploring how to select the best-quality food, we want to emphasize that it is more important to *just start*. While quality matters, letting the pursuit of perfection prevent you from undertaking this journey to wellness is much worse than eating any "less than ideal" foods. See Resources on page 261 for tips on sourcing foods mentioned below.

Meats/Fish

- **GOOD:** If you can't afford or source organic grass-fed or pastured meats or wild-caught seafood, focus on buying leaner cuts of conventionally raised meats (try to make sure they are still hormone-free). Add organ meats and fish to your diet. Conventionally raised organ meat is inexpensive and still very nutrient dense, and farmed fish is better for you than no fish at all. Also consider wild-caught canned salmon, tuna, and sardines, which are cheap, but packed with nutritional value (be sure canned fish is free of soy and spices!). Limit how much conventionally raised poultry you eat, since it has the lowest value in terms of nutrition.

- **BETTER:** If you can afford or source some organic grass-fed or pastured meats or wild-caught seafood, focus on buying fatty cuts. The fat in these animals is great for you! Think fatty roasts and salmon fillets. You might also be able to find high-quality ground meat on sale from time to time. If so, stock up and freeze it.

- **BEST:** Getting all your meat and seafood organic grass-fed or pastured and wild-caught is ideal. Find farmers or fishmon-

gers from whom you can buy directly in bulk in order to save the most money, while getting the highest quality. Ask about buying beef, pork, or lamb in wholes, halves, or quarters. You might be able to share the meat with a group of friends if you don't have enough freezer space or don't have the need for the large quantities. This way, you can take advantage of the lower bulk price and higher quality meat.

Fruits/Vegetables

- **GOOD:** If you cannot get all organic fruits and vegetables, start with the Environmental Working Group's lists of "dirtiest" and "cleanest" produce (see Resources on page 261). These lists are available on their website and published annually, revealing the most pesticide-laden fruits and vegetables versus those that have less chemical residue. These lists are known as the "Dirty Dozen" and the "Clean Fifteen." Focus on avoiding those on the "Dirty Dozen" list. You can also watch for sales on organic, local, in-season produce, as it is usually more economical to buy this way. Finally, check out frozen vegetables. Freezing preserves nutrients and is lower cost.

- **BETTER:** If you can afford some organic produce, focus on organic versions of those on the "Dirty Dozen" list and round out variety with nonorganic fruits and vegetables from the "Clean Fifteen" list. Also, be sure to shop your local farmers' market, looking for great deals on organic, local produce. If you focus on local produce, you may find that your budget can accommodate more than a little organic, since shipping costs are not part of the premium you are paying.

- **BEST:** Get all or as much of your produce as possible organic, local, and in-season. A great way to do this is by joining a CSA with a local farmer. CSA stands for "Community Supported Agriculture." It is when you pay for a share of a farmer's produce at the beginning of a season and then have that share delivered or pick it up weekly during harvest. Fill in variety at the farmers' market, a co-op, or natural food store.

Fats/Oils

- **GOOD:** It is really best to avoid refined vegetable oils as much as possible. If your budget doesn't have a lot of room for high-quality fats and oils, focus on just two staples: coconut oil and olive oil. A fat that is solid at room temperature is best for cooking at high heat. Use the coconut oil for applications like roasting or stir-frying. A fat that is liquid at room temperature is best for cold uses. Use the olive oil for dressings or to drizzle as a topping. Look for the olive oil to be cold-pressed and in an opaque bottle, and buy both in bulk, since it will be much cheaper and you'll be relying on them so much.

- **BETTER:** If you can afford some higher-quality fats and oils, look for pastured animal fats to add to the coconut and olive oil. These fats are solid at room temperature and great for mixing up flavors and nutrients in roasting, stir-frying, etc. If you are willing to render your own lard (pork fat), tallow (beef fat), or duck fat (see page 170), you may be able to purchase large quantities of the fat from a farmer very cheaply. Once rendered, you can store the fat in the refrigerator or freezer. You might also consider adding avocado oil for variety in cold uses.

- **BEST:** The ideal would be purchasing a variety of pastured animal fats (rendering your own or purchasing already rendered), in addition to palm shortening, palm oil, and coconut oil, all of which can be used for high-temperature cooking, plus have different nutritional benefits and flavors. Also have on hand very high quality olive and avocado oil for cold uses.

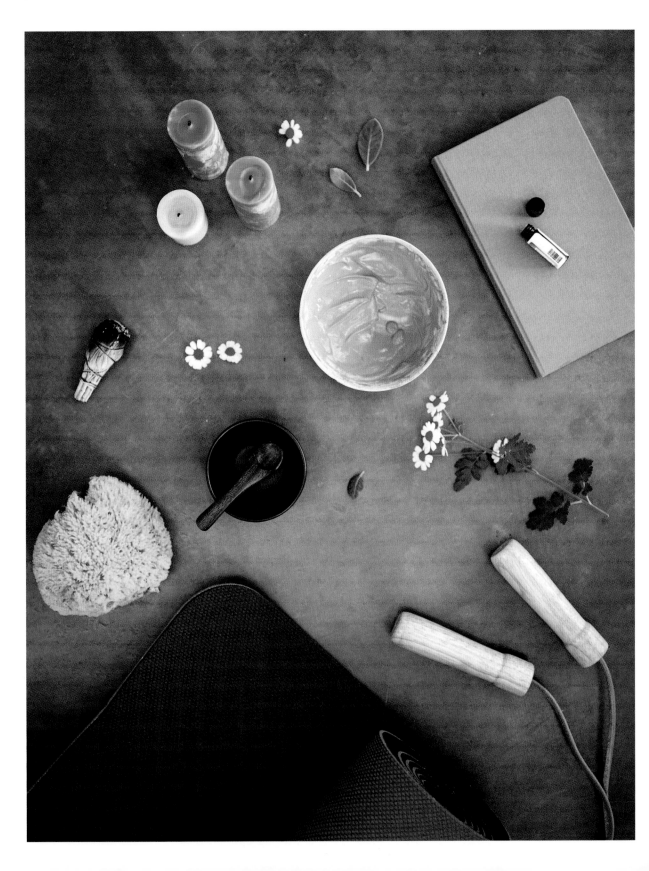

CHAPTER 9

Lifestyle Guide + Exercises

HERE IT IS—THE FINAL PIECE TO putting together a well-rounded life that puts wellness at the top of the list. This is our plan for how to bring all the basic components of sleep, stress management, exercise, and your relationships with others and nature into your life with intention. Not everyone needs to pour himself or herself into every one of these areas—you may have movement handled, but connection is lacking. Others may have strong relationships, but need tons of work on rest. Wherever you are, this plan is laid out to meet your needs and help you take this part of the path to better health many steps further. It is our hope that this wonderful resource will take the burden out of overhauling your habits.

We understand that life with autoimmune disease can leave you feeling incapable of making the smallest change, let alone learning to slow down *and* exercise *and* improve your relationships. When we started to unpack that challenge, we had a realization. A world-class marathoner does not start the race in a sprint. She builds up slowly, so that she can complete the race, rather than burn out early. It is that technique that we've used in designing this plan. You'll find that each step itself is simple, and through a gentle process of layering, you are able to accommodate each change with ease. You don't need a bunch of fancy equipment, and attending a pricey workshop is not required. No trainers, coaches, or mentors are necessary. The preparation list is short and mostly centered on things that are probably already hanging around your house. You have what it takes to start the transformation now!

12-WEEK LIFESTYLE PLAN

When starting this journey to living well with autoimmune disease, it can seem that undertaking dietary changes are the most daunting task. Anyone who has gone through this process for any prolonged period of time will tell you the truth: Lifestyle changes are far and away the hardest to implement. We've found that taking very small, almost micro-size steps is the key. Having a plan that builds over time is not only more achievable, but also more sustainable. You will not realize the benefits of lifestyle changes if you don't practice them over the long-term. With this in mind, we use a 12-week process to build a firm foundation that incorporates all the basics and gives you a chance to try out the many lifestyle suggestions we make in this book. This way, you can discover which routines best support *your* healing process.

Here are a few things to notice about the plan.

- A different area of focus is introduced each week for the first 4 weeks. Week 1 is Rest, Week 2 is Breathe, Week 3 is Move, and Week 4 is Connect.

- At the beginning of each week, you'll have 1 new activity in the 4 areas of Rest, Breathe, Move, or Connect to work on, followed by several days of repeated implementation. For instance, in Week 1 you have 5 days to address how comfortable your bed and bedding are in order to start making small steps to better Rest.

- Weeks 5 through 8 have you taking 1 new step a day in an individual lifestyle area at the beginning of the week, followed by 6 days of tackling all 4 areas for a few minutes at a time. This allows you to slowly adjust your day-to-day schedule in order to accommodate your new focus on overall wellness. We find this is much easier than suddenly being forced to carve out hours you don't have.

- In Weeks 9 through 12, you gradually spend less and less time putting new steps into action and instead put more and more time into the daily practice of *resting, breathing, moving,* and *connecting.* By the end of the 12-week process, with all the basics addressed, you are ready to start fine-tuning your lifestyle to put your health front and center.

We can tell you with confidence—planning and consistent practice are what make long-term lifestyle changes successful. You will notice with each week that these seemingly insignificant actions are building into a dramatic transformation. It is the incentive that will keep you fueled and focused for the journey!

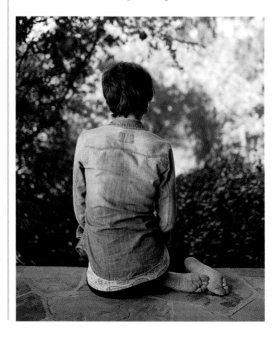

Week 1

	REST	BREATHE	MOVE	CONNECT
MONDAY DAY 1	Do the sleep assessment from page 100 in Chapter 4.	No activity this week	No activity this week	No activity this week
TUESDAY DAY 2	Is your bed and bedding comfortable? If not, use the rest of the week to address this issue.			
WEDNESDAY DAY 3	Comfortable bed/ bedding			
THURSDAY DAY 4	Comfortable bed/ bedding			
FRIDAY DAY 5	Comfortable bed/ bedding			
SATURDAY DAY 6	Comfortable bed/ bedding			
SUNDAY DAY 7	Comfortable bed/ bedding			

If after doing the sleep assessment in Chapter 4, you find that working on Rest is a low priority for you, move on to the Breathe activities in Week 2. If you find that working on Rest is a moderate priority, look ahead at the Rest activities outlined in the plan and focus on the ones that most apply to you. If you find that working on Rest is a high priority, start with Week 1 activities. This week may seem overly slow, even tedious, but take your time.

Week 2

	REST	BREATHE	MOVE	CONNECT
MONDAY DAY 8	Are all the electronics removed from your bedroom? If not, use the rest of this week to address this issue.	Do the stress assessment on page 119 in Chapter 5.	No activity this week	No activity this week
TUESDAY DAY 9	Electronics removed from bedroom	Take the "Identify" step from page 120 of Chapter 5.		
WEDNESDAY DAY 10	Electronics removed from bedroom	5 mins meditation		
THURSDAY DAY 11	Electronics removed from bedroom	5 mins meditation		
FRIDAY DAY 12	Electronics removed from bedroom	5 mins meditation		
SATURDAY DAY 13	Electronics removed from bedroom	5 mins meditation		
SUNDAY DAY 14	Electronics removed from bedroom	5 mins meditation		

If after doing the stress assessment in Chapter 5, you find that working on Breathe activities is a low priority for you, move on to the Move activities in Week 3. If you find that working on Breathe activities is a moderate priority, look ahead at the Breathe activities outlined in the plan and focus on the ones that most apply to you. If you find that working on Breathe activities is a high priority, start with Week 2. You will start meditation this week. Do a little reading online for the best ways to start. Guided meditations, meditative music, or even meditation apps or programs (many of them free) can help you start this practice. It is best if you choose a consistent time each day to do your meditation exercise as well.

Week 3

	REST	BREATHE	MOVE	CONNECT
MONDAY DAY 15	Is your bedroom as dark as possible? If not, use the rest of this week to address this issue.	Take the "Examine" step starting on page 120 of Chapter 5.	Do the exercise assessment on page 143 from Chapter 6.	No activity this week
TUESDAY DAY 16	Dark bedroom	6 mins meditation	Walk for 5 mins today, followed with stretching for 5 mins, for a total of 10 mins.	
WEDNESDAY DAY 17	Dark bedroom	6 mins meditation	10 mins movement	
THURSDAY DAY 18	Dark bedroom	6 mins meditation	10 mins movement	
FRIDAY DAY 19	Dark bedroom	6 mins meditation	10 mins movement	
SATURDAY DAY 20	Dark bedroom	6 mins meditation	10 mins movement	
SUNDAY DAY 21	Dark bedroom	6 mins meditation	10 mins movement	

If after doing the exercise assessment in Chapter 6, you find that working on Move activities is a low priority for you, move on to the Connect activities in Week 4. If you find that working on Move activities is a moderate priority, look at the Move activities outlined in the plan and focus on the ones that most apply to you. If you find that working on Move activities is a high priority, start with Week 3. The easy walking and stretching routine here builds over 10 weeks from extremely minimal activity to a full hour a day. Allow yourself to feel good with the very measured start and don't push ahead too quickly. All you need is a pair of good shoes. Ideas for addressing the darkness of your bedroom are investing in black-out shades, placing duct tape over light sources that can't be removed from your bedroom, or using an eye mask.

Week 4

	REST	BREATHE	MOVE	CONNECT
MONDAY DAY 22	Is your bedroom cool and quiet enough? If not, use the rest of this week to address this issue.	Take the "Eliminate" step from page 122 of Chapter 5.	Walk for 10 mins today, followed with stretching for 5 mins, for a total of 15 mins.	Do the support network assessment on page 151 in Chapter 7.
TUESDAY DAY 23	Cool, quiet bedroom	7 mins meditation	15 mins movement	Look over the "Building a Support Network" section starting on page 150 of Chapter 7. Choose one of those tips to take action on this week.
WEDNESDAY DAY 24	Cool, quiet bedroom	7 mins meditation	15 mins movement	"Building" step
THURSDAY DAY 25	Cool, quiet bedroom	7 mins meditation	15 mins movement	"Building" step
FRIDAY DAY 26	Cool, quiet bedroom	7 mins meditation	15 mins movement	"Building" step
SATURDAY DAY 27	Cool, quiet bedroom	7 mins meditation	15 mins movement	"Building" step
SUNDAY DAY 28	Cool, quiet bedroom	7 mins meditation	15 mins movement	"Building" step

If after doing the support network assessment in Chapter 7, you find that working on Connect activities is a low priority for you, either look ahead at the nature-centered Connect activities outlined in the plan and focus on them or give more energy to the areas of Rest, Breathe, or Move. Ideas for addressing the coolness and quiet of your bedroom are using a fan, setting the thermostat to around 65°F overnight, getting a white noise machine, and/or wearing ear plugs.

The Autoimmune Wellness Handbook

Week 5

	REST	BREATHE	MOVE	CONNECT
MONDAY DAY 29	Have you set a consistent bedtime? If not, use the rest of this week to address this issue.	Take the "Prioritize" step from page 122 of Chapter 5.	Walk for 15 mins today, followed with stretching for 5 mins, for a total of 20 mins.	Look over the "Maintaining Key Support Relationships" section starting on page 152 of Chapter 7. Choose one of those tips to take action on this week.
TUESDAY DAY 30	Consistent bedtime	8 mins meditation	20 mins movement	"Maintaining" step
WEDNESDAY DAY 31	Consistent bedtime	8 mins meditation	20 mins movement	"Maintaining" step
THURSDAY DAY 32	Consistent bedtime	8 mins meditation	20 mins movement	"Maintaining" step
FRIDAY DAY 33	Consistent bedtime	8 mins meditation	20 mins movement	"Maintaining" step
SATURDAY DAY 34	Consistent bedtime	8 mins meditation	20 mins movement	"Maintaining" step
SUNDAY DAY 35	Consistent bedtime	8 mins meditation	20 mins movement	"Maintaining" step

By the fifth week, you'll have worked in each lifestyle area. This week you might want to consider using a pedometer on your walks, if counting steps is motivational for you. In terms of calculating your consistent bedtime, be sure that it gives you a minimum of 8 hours to sleep.

Week 6

	REST	BREATHE	MOVE	CONNECT
MONDAY DAY 36	Do you have a bedtime ritual? If not, use the rest of this week to address this issue.	Take the "Practice" step from page 122 of Chapter 5.	Walk for 20 mins today, followed with stretching for 5 mins, for a total of 25 mins.	Look over the "Addressing Unsupportive Relationships" section starting on page 153 of Chapter 7. Choose one of those tips to take action on this week.
TUESDAY DAY 37	Bedtime ritual	10 mins meditation	25 mins movement	"Addressing" step
WEDNESDAY DAY 38	Bedtime ritual	10 mins meditation	25 mins movement	"Addressing" step
THURSDAY DAY 39	Bedtime ritual	10 mins meditation	25 mins movement	"Addressing" step
FRIDAY DAY 40	Bedtime ritual	10 mins meditation	25 mins movement	"Addressing" step
SATURDAY DAY 41	Bedtime ritual	10 mins meditation	25 mins movement	"Addressing" step
SUNDAY DAY 42	Bedtime ritual	10 mins meditation	25 mins movement	"Addressing" step

You'll note that you are doing 10 whole minutes of a meditation a day now! If you want to do more in the coming weeks, that is fine, but soon we'll start trying other Breathe activities. Ideas for addressing your bedtime ritual are stopping electronic usage 2 to 3 hours before bed, turning down the lights in the house at sunset, using amber-colored glasses before bed, and implementing self-care and calming activities prior to bed.

Week 7

	REST	BREATHE	MOVE	CONNECT
MONDAY DAY 43	Have you set a consistent wake time? If not, use the rest of this week to address this issue.	Take the "Reframe" step from page 122 of Chapter 5.	Walk for 30 mins today, followed with stretching for 10 mins, for a total of 40 mins.	Look over "An Autoimmune-Friendly Social Life" starting on page 154 of Chapter 7. Choose one of those tips to take action on this week.
TUESDAY DAY 44	Consistent wake time	10 mins meditation	40 mins movement	"Social Life" step
WEDNESDAY DAY 45	Consistent wake time	10 mins meditation	40 mins movement	"Social Life" step
THURSDAY DAY 46	Consistent wake time	10 mins meditation	40 mins movement	"Social Life" step
FRIDAY DAY 47	Consistent wake time	10 mins meditation	40 mins movement	"Social Life" step
SATURDAY DAY 48	Consistent wake time	10 mins meditation	40 mins movement	"Social Life" step
SUNDAY DAY 49	Consistent wake time	10 mins meditation	40 mins movement	"Social Life" step

This week, you can continue your 10-minute meditation routine, but you can also now start trying other ways of managing stress. You are also making a big jump this week with the walking and stretching routine. If going from 25 minutes a day to 40 seems to be too much, make a smaller change. You might also consider finding a walking partner this week, since it would be great for *connecting* to others. Listening to podcasts or music while you walk can also enhance your experience. In terms of calculating your consistent wake time, be sure that it gives you a minimum of 8 hours of sleep.

Week 8

	REST	BREATHE	MOVE	CONNECT
MONDAY DAY 50	Do you have a morning ritual? If not, use the rest of this week to address this issue.	Take the "Accept" step from page 123 of Chapter 5.	Walk for 35 mins today, followed with stretching for 10 mins, for a total of 45 mins.	Look at the first two tips in the "How to Start Connecting with Nature" section starting on page 162 of Chapter 7. Choose one of those tips to take action on this week.
TUESDAY DAY 51	Morning ritual	Play	45 mins movement	"Nature" step
WEDNESDAY DAY 52	Morning ritual	Play	45 mins movement	"Nature" step
THURSDAY DAY 53	Morning ritual	Play	45 mins movement	"Nature" step
FRIDAY DAY 54	Morning ritual	Play	45 mins movement	"Nature" step
SATURDAY DAY 55	Morning ritual	Play	45 mins movement	"Nature" step
SUNDAY DAY 56	Morning ritual	Play	45 mins movement	"Nature" step

The Breathe activity this week is to try play. If active play does not seem doable for you, try coloring, playing with clay, or building with Legos. Remember how you liked playing as a child, and give it a shot. You'll also begin Connect activities that emphasize nature. Don't discount the power of this step. Ideas for addressing your morning ritual are getting outside first thing in order to get exposure to sunlight or investing in a light-therapy lamp in order to start signaling your brain to produce the correct hormones.

The Autoimmune Wellness Handbook

Week 9

	REST	BREATHE	MOVE	CONNECT
MONDAY DAY 57	If you are continuing to struggle with sleep, consider talking with your health-care provider. Use the rest of this month to troubleshoot.	Begin working on the "Alter" step, if necessary, from page 123 of Chapter 5.	Walk for 40 mins today, followed with stretching for 10 mins, for a total of 50 mins.	Look at the third tip in the "How to Start Connecting with Nature" section starting on page 162 of Chapter 7. Consider small changes to take action on this week.
TUESDAY DAY 58	Troubleshoot sleep	Journal	50 mins movement	"Indoor" step
WEDNESDAY DAY 59	Troubleshoot sleep	Journal	50 mins movement	"Indoor" step
THURSDAY DAY 60	Troubleshoot sleep	Journal	50 mins movement	"Indoor" step
FRIDAY DAY 61	Troubleshoot sleep	Journal	50 mins movement	"Indoor" step
SATURDAY DAY 62	Troubleshoot sleep	Journal	50 mins movement	"Indoor" step
SUNDAY DAY 63	Troubleshoot sleep	Journal	50 mins. movement	"Indoor" step

This week, you'll see that you've taken all the basic steps with Rest and can start troubleshooting any remaining sleep problems with your key player, if this area continues to be problematic for you. You'll also start working on altering, if necessary, any areas of your life that are major sources of stress that were not successfully addressed using other steps. This could potentially be a huge process and should be undertaken with the support of your health-care team, including a therapist.

Week 10

	REST	BREATHE	MOVE	CONNECT
MONDAY DAY 64	Troubleshoot sleep	If the "Alter" step was necessary, you may still need time to work on this step.	Walk for 50 mins today, followed with stretching for 10 mins, for a total of 60 mins.	Look at the fourth tip in the "How to Start Connecting with Nature" section on page 163 of Chapter 7. Start planning a 2- to 3-hour nature day trip.
TUESDAY DAY 65	Troubleshoot sleep	Listen to music	60 mins movement	"Day Trip" step
WEDNESDAY DAY 66	Troubleshoot sleep	Listen to music	60 mins movement	"Day Trip" step
THURSDAY DAY 67	Troubleshoot sleep	Listen to music	60 mins movement	"Day Trip" step
FRIDAY DAY 68	Troubleshoot sleep	Listen to music	60 mins movement	"Day Trip" step
SATURDAY DAY 69	Troubleshoot sleep	Listen to music	60 mins movement	"Day Trip" step
SUNDAY DAY 70	Troubleshoot sleep	Listen to music	60 mins movement	"Day Trip" step

If altering any area of your life to better manage stress was necessary, from this point forward, you may need a great deal of time to troubleshoot how to make those changes. That said, there are still daily things you can try to help manage stress. In addition to your 10-minute meditation routine, you might try listening to music this week. You've also reached a full hour of activity a day! Finally, you'll start working on how to spend 2 to 3 hours weekly just soaking in the natural environment.

The Autoimmune Wellness Handbook

Week 11

	REST	BREATHE	MOVE	CONNECT
MONDAY DAY 71	Troubleshoot sleep	Try massage or acupuncture	Start finding ways to increase movement at your workplace and throughout your day.	Look at the fifth tip in the "How to Start Connecting with Nature" section on page 163 of Chapter 7. Start planning a 2-day nature trip.
TUESDAY DAY 72	Troubleshoot sleep	Try massage or acupuncture	Increase movement	"2-Day Trip" step
WEDNESDAY DAY 73	Troubleshoot sleep	Try massage or acupuncture	Increase movement	"2-Day Trip" step
THURSDAY DAY 74	Troubleshoot sleep	Try massage or acupuncture	Increase movement	"2-Day Trip" step
FRIDAY DAY 75	Troubleshoot sleep	Try massage or acupuncture	Increase movement	"2-Day Trip" step
SATURDAY DAY 76	Troubleshoot sleep	Try massage or acupuncture	Increase movement	"2-Day Trip" step
SUNDAY DAY 77	Troubleshoot sleep	Try massage or acupuncture	Increase movement	"2-Day Trip" step

A big step this week in terms of Breathe activities will be to try out something like massage or acupuncture. You'll also start thinking about new ways to increase exercise in your life and how to increase your time in nature with a 2-day trip. Involve friends and family in this plan; make it fun to discover how nature impacts your wellness.

Week 12

	REST	BREATHE	MOVE	CONNECT
MONDAY DAY 78	Troubleshoot sleep	Try mindfulness	Increase movement	If you've been working on a 2-day nature trip, you may still need time to work on this step.
TUESDAY DAY 79	Troubleshoot sleep	Try mindfulness	Increase movement	"2-Day Trip" step
WEDNESDAY DAY 80	Troubleshoot sleep	Try mindfulness	Increase movement	"2-Day Trip" step
THURSDAY DAY 81	Troubleshoot sleep	Try mindfulness	Increase movement	"2-Day Trip" step
FRIDAY DAY 82	Troubleshoot sleep	Try mindfulness	Increase movement	Fine-tune lifestyle according to your preferences, budget, and needs in order to maximize wellness.
SATURDAY DAY 83	Troubleshoot sleep	Try mindfulness	Increase movement	"Fine-Tune" step
SUNDAY DAY 84	Troubleshoot sleep	Try mindfulness	Increase movement	"Fine-Tune" step

You have reached the end of the process and brought all the basics into your new wellness lifestyle. From here on, this process is about fine-tuning according to your preferences, budget, and changing needs, so that you can maximize living well with autoimmune disease.

LIFESTYLE PLAN PREPARATION LIST

Here is a list of all of the tools and supplies you may need in order to follow the 12-Week Lifestyle Plan, arranged in 4-week blocks. None of them is unusual, but it is helpful to make sure you have everything you need before getting started. We've also included a list of optional items, which make some activities easier. For product recommendations for some of these tools and supplies, see Resources on page 261.

Weeks 1–4

- Pen and paper for taking assessments and doing the Breathe activities
- Timer for timing meditation and exercise routines
- Walking shoes for exercise routines

Optional (you'll only need these if you find they have to be addressed for proper Rest or Breathe activities)

- New bed and/or bedding
- Black-out shades, duct tape, eye mask
- Ear plugs, white noise machine, fan
- Guided meditations, meditation music, or meditation apps/programs

Weeks 5–8

- Clock for noting consistent bedtimes and wake times
- Journal
- Play items (coloring books, colored pencils, clay, Legos, etc.)

Optional (you'll only need these if you find they have to be addressed for proper Rest or Move activities)

- Amber glasses
- Light-therapy lamp
- Pedometer
- iPod/headphones

Weeks 9–12

- No new materials are required at this point.

Optional (you'll only need these if you find they have to be addressed for proper Move or Connect activities)

- Backpack and water bottle
- Camping gear
- Houseplants
- Essential oils

Conclusion: Putting It All Together

IMPLEMENTING THE CHANGES WE TALK ABOUT in this book will take time and persistence. This undertaking does not happen in weeks or even months—both of us have been engaging in this process for many years now and are *continuing* to troubleshoot and edit, as necessary. The beauty of adopting a diet and lifestyle *template* instead of a *prescription* is that you can adjust your habits and routines based on the ebb and flow of your changing daily life. In times of high stress or flare, you "batten down the hatches." You tighten your approach to the diet and lifestyle aspects of this process in order to restore balance. In times of ease or good health, you "unfurl the sails." You embrace a more expansive approach that allows you to enjoy, experiment, and experience the boundaries of wellness with autoimmune disease. This is what the ebb and flow will eventually look like, but, in the beginning, you need to methodically follow the process, from start to finish.

In this book, we've presented you with seven powerful steps on the autoimmune wellness journey: *inform, collaborate, nourish, rest, breathe, move,* and *connect.* In addition to a wealth of information to guide your actions, we've given you all the tools and resources you need to get started, like meal plans, recipes, a lifestyle guide, and self-assessments. These changes, while powerful on their own, are synergistic and combine to form a comprehensive approach that will revolutionize your healing process. Gradually, you will learn how to integrate the best of medical care with these DIY modifications. Using the tools presented here to define your personal priorities on this journey will help you pinpoint which actions are going to be most transformative for you. Having walked this path ourselves, our goal is to make this process easier and more actionable.

One important thing we want to emphasize as we come to the end of our time together, is that perfectionism has no part in this process. Let go of the need to do it all right straight out of the gate. Take this slowly, patiently putting one foot in front of the other. If you hit a stumbling block, reevaluate, regroup, and move forward with your new knowledge. It's not about doing everything perfectly; it is about understanding that effort over time will produce change. Water cuts through rock and makes its way to the sea not by knowing the exact route, but through persistence over time.

When we started to make these changes in our own lives, to be honest, the information overload made it feel like we were drinking from a fire hose. This process is unfamiliar and uncomfortable at the start. We've been in your shoes! Our culture makes these dietary and lifestyle modifications more difficult; by choosing to heal in this way, you will be going against the stream. You are taking responsibility for your health in a society that says, "Just take a pill . . . and stop for fast food on the way home from the pharmacy." From that perspective, you realize that the adjustment here is not just about reorganizing your schedule or your kitchen or your food budget . . . it's also about shifting what you see as normal. It is okay to have some meltdowns, because, in all honesty, this is going to be one of the harder things you've ever done.

We're here to tell you *it really does get easier with time!* You'll have it wired soon, and, as healing takes hold and energy returns, you won't believe you thought that any other way was normal. Hang in there! There is a growing community of people who are undertaking these changes and shifting the way autoimmune disease recovery is achieved. If we didn't believe it was worth it, if we had not experienced incredible healing ourselves, if we had not watched hundreds of other people experi-

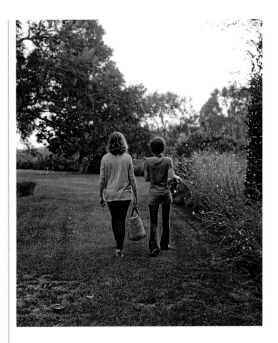

ence the same, we would not have tackled this project!

The final chapter of this book marks the next chapter of your life with autoimmune disease—one that is filled with empowerment, action, wellness, and vitality. You are likely to uncover a part of yourself that you didn't know existed. Our hope is that the tools and resources found in this book will help you make informed, practical choices, and that, once your health is restored, you will add your voice to the revolutionary shift that is under way in the autoimmune community. We invite you to take ownership of your journey and join us in pioneering this new era. This is wellness that outlasts the hype!

Gratitude

David Alt and Maggee Hunt, for loving me delicately, but expecting me to be as tough as nails.

Noah Trescott, for giving so much of yourself so that I could complete this project. I could not have made it without your service, insight, and tough love.

Charlotte Dupont, for her unique, inspiring photography. Your touch adds depth to this project that we could not communicate with words. Thanks for waking up whimsical.

Rose Sullivan, Brian Sullivan, Lori Miller, and Gary and Lynnette Clark, for supporting us as we won back our health and through the journey of writing another book.

Sarah Ballantyne, for her research and development of the Autoimmune Protocol, as well as for allowing us to use it in this book. Your work changed our lives and inspires us daily to spread the word.

Terry Wahls, Robb Wolf, and Chris Kresser, for providing valuable, accessible information that has transformed not only our lives, but many other lives, and helped inform this book.

Grace Heerman, for managing our work tasks and social media while writing this book. We are so proud to have you on our team!

The Pulice family, for generously allowing us to cook and take photographs for our book at their beautiful ranch. We wanted to communicate healing, and your home is overflowing with it.

Celeste Fine and John Maas, for their representation and support throughout this process. We are grateful for your professional guidance.

Marisa Vigilante and her team at Rodale, for helping us create a book that would accurately convey the depth of our passion and be a valuable tool for others.

Yrmis Barroeta, Bobby Chang, Moya Chang, Titus Chiu, Natasha Fallahi, Susan McCauley, Felix Madrid, Stephanie Madrid, Mary Cloos, Katie Sullivan, Rose Sullivan, Jason Handler, Stacy Pulice, Jordan, and Amanda, for modeling for us and participating in photo shoots for the book.

The community of Autoimmune Protocol bloggers, for collaborating with us to write about autoimmune hope and healing. We count ourselves lucky to be changing the world with people like you.

Our readers and supporters, for being willing to try a whole new approach to wellness. You have energized this project and motivate us daily. Without your enthusiasm, this book would not have been possible.

Resources

AUTOIMMUNE DISEASE ORGANIZATIONS

American Autoimmune Related Diseases Organization www.aarda.org

Arthritis Foundation www.arthritis.org

Celiac Disease Foundation www.celiac.org

Crohn's and Colitis Foundation of America www.ccfa.org

Endometriosis.org www.endometriosis.org

Graves' Disease and Thyroid Foundation www.gdatf.org

Hashimoto's Awareness www.hashimotosawareness.org

International Foundation for Autoimmune Arthritis www.ifautoimmunearthritis.org

Lupus and Allied Diseases Association www.nolupus.org

Lupus Foundation of America www.lupus.org

Myasthenia Gravis Foundation of America, Inc. www.myasthenia.org

The Myositis Association www.myositis.org

National Alopecia Areata Foundation www.naaf.org

National Multiple Sclerosis Society www.nationalmssociety.org

National Psoriasis Foundation www.psoriasis.org

Platelet Disorder Support Association www.pdsa.org

Scleroderma Foundation www.scleroderma.org

Sjögrens Syndrome Foundation www.sjogrens.org

Thyroid Change www.thyroidchange.org

AUTOIMMUNE PROTOCOL ONLINE RESOURCES

Autoimmune Paleo www.autoimmune-paleo.com

The Paleo Mom www.thepaleomom.com

Phoenix Helix www.phoenixhelix.com

AUTOIMMUNE PROTOCOL RECIPE BOOKS

The Alternative Autoimmune Cookbook by Angie Alt with Jenifer Beehler

The Autoimmune Paleo Cookbook by Mickey Trescott, NTP

The Healing Kitchen by Alaena Haber, MS, OTR, and Sarah Ballantyne, PhD

He Won't Know It's Paleo by Bre'anna Emmitt

Nourish by Rachael Bryant

The Paleo Approach Cookbook by Sarah Ballantyne, PhD

Simple French Paleo by Sophie Van Tiggelen

CONNECT

Autoimmune Protocol Meetup Groups www.autoimmune-paleo.com/meetup

Discover the Forest www.discoverthefores.org

National Park Foundation www.nationalparks.org

National Park Service www.findyourpark.com

The Wilderness Society www.wilderness.org

FINDING A DOCTOR

Academy of Integrative Health and Medicine
www.aihm.org

The American Association of Naturopathic
Physicians www.naturopathic.org

American Board of Integrative Holistic Medicine
www.abihm.org/search-doctors

American College for Advancement in Medicine
www.acam.org

Canadian Association of Naturopathic Doctors
www.cand.ca

The Institute for Functional Medicine
www.functionalmedicine.org

International College of Integrative Medicine
www.icimed.com

Paleo Physicians Network
www.paleophysiciansnetwork.com

Primal Docs www.primaldocs.com

Revive Primary Care www.reviveprimarycare.com

FOOD SOURCING

Azure Standard of Healthy and Abundant
Living www.azurestandard.com

Eat Wild www.eatwild.com

Environmental Working Group www.ewg.org

LocalFarmMarkets.org
www.localfarmmarkets.org

Local Harvest www.localharvest.org

National Farmers Market Directory
www.nfmd.org

Thrive Market www.thrivemarket.com

US Wellness Meats www.grasslandbeef.com

Vital Choice Wild Seafood and Organics
www.vitalchoice.com/shop/pc/home.asp

Wild Fermentation www.wildfermentation.com

FURTHER READING

Adrenal Fatigue by James Wilson, ND, DC, PhD

The Autoimmune Solution by Amy Myers, MD

Digestive Health with Real Food by Aglaée
Jacob, MS, RD

Hashimoto's Thyroiditis by Izabella Wentz,
PharmD, FASCP

The Hidden Plague by Tara Grant

Move Your DNA by Katy Bowman, MS

The Paleo Approach by Sarah Ballantyne, PhD

The Paleo Solution by Robb Wolf

The Wahls Protocol by Terry Wahls, MD

*Why Do I Still Have Thyroid Symptoms? When
My Lab Tests Are Normal* by Datis
Kharrazian, DHSc, DC, MS

Why Isn't My Brain Working? by Datis
Kharrazian, DHSc, DC, MS

You're Not Crazy and You're Not Alone by
Stacey Robbins

Your Personal Paleo Code by Chris Kresser

INGREDIENTS/SNACKS

Artisan Tropic www.artisantropic.com

Bare Bones www.barebonesbroth.com

Bragg www.bragg.com

Coconut Secret www.coconutsecret.com
/index.html

Edward and Sons www.edwardandsons.com

EPIC www.epicbar.com

Fatworks www.fatworksfoods.com

Great Lakes Gelatin www.greatlakesgelatin.com

Jackson's Honest www.jacksonshonest.com

Kasadrinos www.kasandrinos.com

McCormick Gourmet www.mccormick.com
/gourmet

Mission Heirloom www.missionheirloom.com

Natural Value www.naturalvalue.com/product
/organic-coconut-milk

Nutiva www.nutiva.com

Otto's Naturals www.ottosnaturals.com

Our Amazon store www.autoimmune-paleo.com
/amazon

Paleo Angel www.paleoangel.com

The Pure Wraps www.thepurewraps.com

Real Salt www.realsalt.com

Red Boat Fish Sauce www.redboatfishsauce.com

Salt, Fire, and Time www.saltfireandtime.com

Seasnax www.seasnax.com

Tropical Traditions www.tropicaltraditions.com

Vital Proteins www.vitalproteins.com

KITCHEN TOOLS

Bamboo spoons www.autoimmune-paleo.com
/bamboospoons

Berkey Filters www.berkeyfilters.com

Cuisinart www.cuisinart.com

GIR spatula www.productofgir.com

Gummy molds www.autoimmune-paleo.com
/gelatinmolds

Instant Pot www.instantpot.com

Lodge Cast Iron www.lodgemfg.com

Spiralizer www.autoimmune-paleo.com
/spiralizer

ThermoWorks www.thermoworks.com

Vitamix www.vitamix.com

MOVEMENT

Altra www.altrarunning.com

Body image www.theperformingwoman.com

ReboundAir www.rebound-air.com

Vivobarefoot www.vivobarefoot.com

SLEEP

Air purifier www.autoimmune-paleo.com
/airpurifier

Ambient noise machine www.autoimmune
-paleo.com/noisemachine

Blue-light blocking glasses
www.autoimmune-paleo.com/blueblockers

Blue-light blocking software www.justgetflux
.com

Light therapy lamp
www.autoimmune-paleo.com/therapylamp

STRESS MANAGEMENT

Headspace www.headspace.com

Mountain Rose Herbs
www.mountainroseherbs.com

Resilience Academy www.resilienceacademy.com

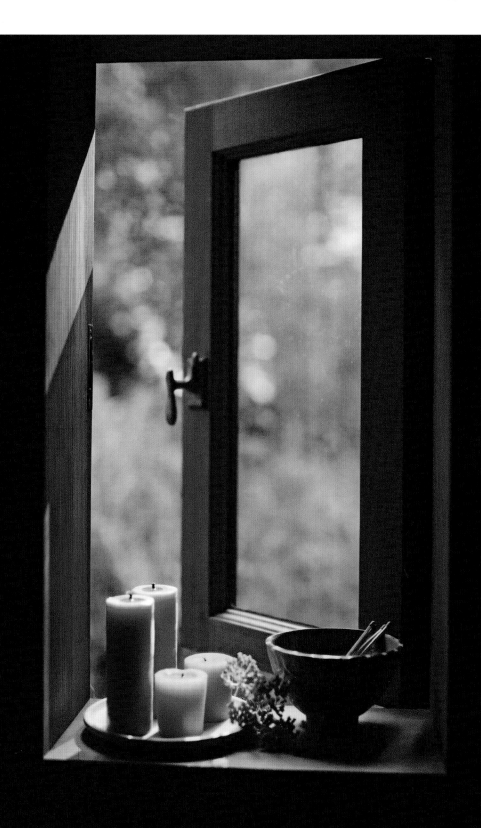

References

Chapter 1

* www.aarda.org/autoimmune-information/autoimmune-statistics
* www.ncbi.nlm.nih.gov/pmc/articles/PMC3384703
* www.ncbi.nlm.nih.gov/pmc/articles/PMC3458511
* womenshealth.gov/publications/our-publications/fact-sheet/autoimmune-diseases.html#a
* www.nlm.nih.gov/medlineplus/ency/article/000816.htm
* www.niams.nih.gov/health_info/autoimmune/
* www.autoimmune.pathology.jhmi.edu/whatis_disease.cfm
* www.drhyman.com/blog/2010/07/30/how-to-stop-attacking-yourself-9-steps-to-heal-autoimmune-disease/
* www.cancer.org/cancer/cancerbasics/cancer-prevalence
* www.diabetesed.net/page/_files/autoimmune-diseases.pdf
* www.books.nap.edu/openbook.php?record_id=12908
* www.aarda.org/autoimmune-information/autoimmune-disease-in-women/
* www.report.nih.gov/categorical_spending.aspx
* www.aarda.org/autoimmune-information/questions-and-answers/
* www.autoimmune.pathology.jhmi.edu/whatisautoimmunity.cfm
* www.medscape.com/viewarticle/449854_11
* www.usa.healthcare.siemens.com/clinical-specialities/womens-health-information/laboratory-diagnostics/autoimmune-disorders
* www.everydayhealth.com/autoimmune-disorders/autoimmune-risk-factors.aspx
* www.benaroyaresearch.org/what-is-bri/disease-information/autoimmune-diseases#.VXg4K6aHjd5
* www.elaine-moore.com/Articles/AutoimmuneDiseases/MultipleAutoimmuneSyndrome/tabid/229/Default.aspx
* www.ncbi.nlm.nih.gov/pmc/articles/PMC3150011/
* *The Paleo Approach* by Sarah Ballantyne, PhD, p. 42.
* www.celiacdisease.about.com/od/faqs/f/Celiac-Testing-Relatives.htm

* *The Paleo Approach* by Sarah Ballantyne, PhD, pp. 17–19.

* www.aarda.org/autoimmune
-information/list-of-diseases/

* www.aarda.org/wp-content/uploads
/2013/08/tips_for_auto_diagnosis.pdf

* www.mindbodygreen.com/0-8843
/10-signs-you-have-an-autoimmune
-disease-how-to-reverse-it.html

* www.womenshealth.gov/publications
/our-publications/fact-sheet
/autoimmune-diseases.html

* www.diabetesed.net/page/_files
/autoimmune-diseases.pdf

* www.aarda.org/wp-content/uploads
/2013/08/tips_for_auto_diagnosis.pdf

* www.celiaccentral.org/celiac-disease
/facts-and-figures

* www.mollysfund.org/2013/04/lupus
-overlap-diseases-what-are-some
-common-diseases-associated-with
-lupus

* www.ncbi.nlm.nih.gov/pubmed
/20103030

* www.msfocus.org/article-details
.aspx?articleID=18

* www.grief.com/the-five-stages-of
-grief/

* www.hss.edu/conditions_who-am-i
-now-living-with-autoimmune
-disease.asp#.VYBHH6aHjd4

* www.aarda.org/wp-content/uploads
/2013/11/Families-Coping-with
-Autoimmune-Disease.pdf

* www.psychologytoday.com/blog/the
-squeaky-wheel/201501/how-coping
-chronic-illness-impacts-loneliness

* www.time.com/3702101/navy-seal
-secrets-grit-resilience/

* www.time.com/3892044/the-science
-of-bouncing-back

* www.everydayhealth.com
/autoimmune-disorders/autoimmune
-disorders-and-your-emotional
-health.aspx

* www.my.clevelandclinic.org/health
/healthy_living/hic_Stress
_Management_and_Emotional
_Health/hic_Fostering_a_Positive
_Self-Image

* www.nlm.nih.gov/medlineplus/ency
/article/000816.htm

* www.celiaccentral.org/gettested/

* www.celiaccentral.org/followup/

* www.rheumatology.org/Practice
/Clinical/Patients/Diseases_And
_Conditions/Rheumatoid_Arthritis/

* www.ncbi.nlm.nih.gov/pmc/articles
/PMC3683194/

* www.nationalmssociety.org
/Symptoms-Diagnosis/Diagnosing
-Tools/MRI

* www.mayoclinic.org/tests
-procedures/endoscopy/basics
/definition/prc-20020363

* www.mayoclinic.org/tests
-procedures/colonoscopy/basics
/definition/prc-20013624

- www.mayoclinic.org/tests -procedures/x-ray/basics/definition /prc-20009519
- www.mayoclinic.org/tests -procedures/ultrasound/basics /definition/prc-20020341
- www.rheumatology.org/Practice /Clinical/Patients/Diseases_And _Conditions/Antinuclear_Antibodies _(ANA)/
- www.mayoclinic.org/thyroid-disease /expert-answers/faq-20058114
- www.mayoclinic.org/tests -procedures/complete-blood-count /basics/definition/prc-20014088
- www.mayoclinic.org/tests -procedures/c-reactive-protein /basics/definition/prc-20014480
- www.functionalmedicine.org/files /library/experience-life-functional.pdf
- www.aarda.org/autoimmune -information/questions-and-answers/
- www.arthritis.org/about-arthritis /types/rheumatoid-arthritis /treatment.php
- www.ccfa.org/what-are-crohns-and -colitis/what-is-crohns-disease /crohns-treatment-options.html ?referrer=https://www.google.com/
- www.my.clevelandclinic.org/health /drugs_devices_supplements/hic _Non-Steroidal_Anti-Inflammatory _Medicines_NSAIDs
- www.mayoclinic.org/steroids/art -20045692

- www.ncbi.nlm.nih.gov/pubmed /17458395
- www.ncbi.nlm.nih.gov/pmc/articles /PMC2592779/
- www.rheumatology.oxfordjournals .org/content/51/suppl_6/vi37.full
- www.rightdiagnosis.com/a/ai /prognosis.htm
- www.merckmanuals.com/home /immune-disorders/allergic -reactions-and-other-hypersensitivity -disorders/autoimmune-disorders

Chapter 2

- www.nursingworld.org/MainMenu Categories/ANAMarketplace/ANA Periodicals/OJIN/TableofContents /Volume102005/No1Jan05/tpc26 _116008.aspx
- *Ten Lessons in Collaboration* (presentation) by Deborah B. Gardner, PhD.
- www.nlm.nih.gov/medlineplus/ency /article/001933.htm
- www.osteopathic.org/osteopathic -health/about-dos/what-is-a-do /Pages/default.aspx
- www.aanp.org/all-about-nps/what -is-an-np
- www.nccpa.net/public
- www.naturopathic.org/content.asp ?contentid=59
- www.ccaom.org/faqs.asp
- www.moveforwardpt.com/AboutPTs PTAs/Default.aspx#.VYw47BNVhBc

* www.amtamassage.org
  /findamassage/credential.html

* www.altmedworld.net/alternative.htm

* www.healthandhealingny.org
  /complement/homeo_training.html

* www.reiki.org/FAQ/WhatIsReiki.html

* www.functionalmedicine.org/about
  /whatisfm/

* www.nccih.nih.gov/health
  /integrative-health

* www.nationalpartnership.org
  /research-library/health-care
  /petm-presenter-manual.pdf

* www.nursingworld.org/MainMenu
  Categories/ANAMarketplace/ANA
  Periodicals/OJIN/TableofContents
  /Volume102005/No1Jan05/tpc26
  _116008.aspx

* www.quickanddirtytips.com/health
  -fitness/prevention/how-to-find-a
  -good-primary-care-doctor?page=1

* www.pamfblog.org/2011/06
  /choosing-a-primary-care-doctor/

* www.bcbs.com/blog/five-tips-for
  -choosing-a-PCP.html

* www.nationalpartnership.org
  /research-library/health-care
  /petm-presenter-manual.pdf

* www.cfah.org/prepared-patient
  /prepared-patient-articles/giving
  -your-doctor-the-pink-slip

* www.health.usnews.com/top-doctors
  /articles/2011/07/26/9-signs-you
  -should-fire-your-doctor

* *The Wahls Protocol* by Terry Wahls,
  MD, pp. 261–64.

Chapter 3

* www.gut.bmj.com/content/49/2/159
  .long

* *The Paleo Approach* by Sarah
  Ballantyne, PhD, p. 53.

* www.jcs.biologists.org/content/113
  /24/4435.abstract?ijkey=130db389d2
  00d07d6f48e9d3651c3f0e868b78f4&k
  eytype2=tf_ipsecsha

* www.ncbi.nlm.nih.gov/pmc/articles
  /PMC3384703

* www.physrev.physiology.org/content
  /91/1/151.long

* www.ncbi.nlm.nih.gov/pmc/articles
  /PMC3458511

* www.link.springer.com/article/10
  .1007%2Fs12016-011-8291-x

* www.healthline.com/health/gerd
  /statistics

* www.ncbi.nlm.nih.gov/pmc/articles
  /PMC2974811

* www.well.blogs.nytimes.com/2012
  /06/25/combating-acid-reflux-may
  -bring-host-of-ills/?_r=0

* www.ncbi.nlm.nih.gov/pmc/articles
  /PMC3098920

* www.ncbi.nlm.nih.gov/pmc/articles
  /PMC3820047/

* www.cghjournal.org/article/S1542
  -3565(15)00153-6/fulltext

* *The Paleo Approach* by Sarah
  Ballantyne, PhD, pp. 185–86.

* www.foodallergy.org/diagnosis-and
  -testing/oral-food-challenge
* *The Paleo Approach* by Sarah
  Ballantyne, PhD, pp.
* www.chriskresser.com/pills-or
  -paleo-preventing-and-reversing
  -autoimmune-disease/
* www.thepaleomom.com
  /autoimmunity/the-autoimmune
  -protocol
* *The Paleo Approach* by Sarah
  Ballantyne, PhD, Ch 5.
* www.marksdailyapple.com/cold
  -turkey-vs-baby-steps-which-is-the
  -better-approach/#axzz3fCRy3aLP
* *The Paleo Approach* by Sarah
  Ballantyne, PhD, Ch. 9.
* www.eatingdisorderhope.com/
* www.allianceforeatingdisorders
  .com/portal/home
* www.nationaleatingdisorders.org
* www./radicatamedicine.files
  .wordpress.com/2014/06/paleo
  -fodmap-food-list.pdf
* *Digestive Health with Real Food* by
  Aglaée Jacob
* www.ajcn.nutrition.org/content/85
  /5/1185.full.pdf+html
* www.ajcn.nutrition.org/content/85
  /5/1185/T3.expansion.html

Chapter 4

* *Your Personal Paleo Code* by Chris
  Kresser, pp. 227–28.
* www.cdc.gov/features/dssleep

* *The Paleo Approach* by Sarah
  Ballantyne, PhD, pp. 255–58.
* www.chriskresser.com/beyond
  -paleo-9
* www.ncbi.nlm.nih.gov/pubmed
  /26197315
* www.chriskresser.com/how-much
  -sleep-do-you-need
* www.ajpregu.physiology.org/content
  /ajpregu/246/2/R161.full.pdf
* www.anapsid.org/cnd/files/sleep-in
  -selected-ai.pdf
* www.chriskresser.com/ask-the-rd
  -nutrition-for-better-sleep-and
  -gaining-weight-on-paleo/
* *Your Personal Paleo Code* by Chris
  Kesser, pp. 227–36, 243–45, 228–37.
* *The Paleo Approach* by Sarah
  Ballantyne, PhD, pp. 131, 144–57,
  151–53, 157, 257.
* www.sleepfoundation.org

Chapter 5

* *Your Personal Paleo Code* by Chris
  Kresser, pp. 241–45.
* *The Paleo Approach* by Sarah
  Ballantyne, PhD, pp. 246–49.
* www.explorable.com/general
  -adaptation-syndrome
* www.apa.org/news/press/releases
  /2007/10/stress.aspx
* www.apa.org/news/press/releases
  /stress/2014
* www.mayoclinic.org/healthy
  -lifestyle/stress-management
  /in-depth/stress/art-20046037

- www.helpguide.org/articles/stress /stress-management.htm
- *Adrenal Fatigue* by James L. Wilson, ND, DC, PhD, pp. 104–7.
- *David and Goliath* by Malcolm Gladwell, p. 102.

Chapter 6

- www.apocpcontrol.org/paper_file /issue_abs/Volume8_No3/325- 338%20b_Kruk14.pdf
- www.download.springer.com/static /pdf/331/art%253A10.1007%25 2Fs40279-015-0363-2.pdf?originUrl =http%3A%2F%2Flink.springer.com %2Farticle%2F10.1007%2Fs40279 -015-0363-2&token2=exp=1438613838 ~acl=%2Fstatic%2Fpdf%2F331%2Fart %25253A10.1007%25252Fs40279-015 -0363-2.pdf%3ForiginUrl%3Dhttp %253A%252F%252Flink.springer.com %252Farticle%252F10.1007%25 2Fs40279-015-0363-2*~hmac =a93c680d67b2fef5bbf85b6711f d484087e40ef44cd4a3e4804afca 9660b4856
- www.mdpi.com/1422-0067/16/7 /14901/htm
- www.circ.ahajournals.org/content /107/1/e2.full
- www.cdc.gov/physicalactivity/data /facts.htm
- *The Paleo Approach* by Sarah Ballantyne, PhD, pp. 158–62.
- *Your Personal Paleo Code* by Chris Kresser, p. 120.
- www.inmyskinnygenes.com/2013 /10/21/disgust-body-shame-and -fitspiration-maria-kang/
- www.ncbi.nlm.nih.gov/pmc/articles /PMC4389710/
- *The Paleo Approach* by Sarah Ballantyne, PhD, pp. 258–59.
- *Your Personal Paleo Code* by Chris Kresser, pp. 214–15.
- www.ncbi.nlm.nih.gov/pmc/articles /PMC3098122/
- www.well.blogs.nytimes.com/2014 /04/30/want-to-be-more-creative -take-a-walk/?_r=2
- www.scientificamerican.com/article /regular-walking-can-help-ease -depression
- www.well.blogs.nytimes.com/2013 /08/12/building-up-bones-with-a -little-bashing
- www.health.howstuffworks.com /wellness/diet-fitness/exercise /benefits-of-walking5.htm
- www.ncbi.nlm.nih.gov/pubmed /21364350

Chapter 7

- *Social: Why Our Brains Are Wired to Connect* by Matthew D. Lieberman, pp. 39–70.
- *Your Personal Paleo Code* by Chris Kresser, pp. 262–63.
- www.thepaleomom.com/2014/12 /health-benefits-connection.html

* www.heretohelp.bc.ca/sites/default /files/wellness-module-3-social -support.pdf

* www.psychologytoday.com/blog /compassion-matters/201301/5-ways -maintain-lifelong-friendships

* www.psychcentral.com/lib/why -friends-disappear-when-crisis -turns-chronic/

* *Your Personal Paleo Code* by Chris Kresser, pp. 271–73.

* www.jameslovelock.org/page34.html

* www.ncbi.nlm.nih.gov/pmc/articles /PMC2793347

* www.ncbi.nlm.nih.gov/pmc/articles /PMC2793341

* www.ncbi.nlm.nih.gov/pmc/articles /PMC2793346

* www.ncbi.nlm.nih.gov/pmc/articles /PMC3699874

* www.ncbi.nlm.nih.gov/pmc/articles /PMC3987044

* www.ncbi.nlm.nih.gov/pmc/articles /PMC4276610/#B1-ijerph-11-12204

* www.ncbi.nlm.nih.gov/pmc/articles /PMC4233975

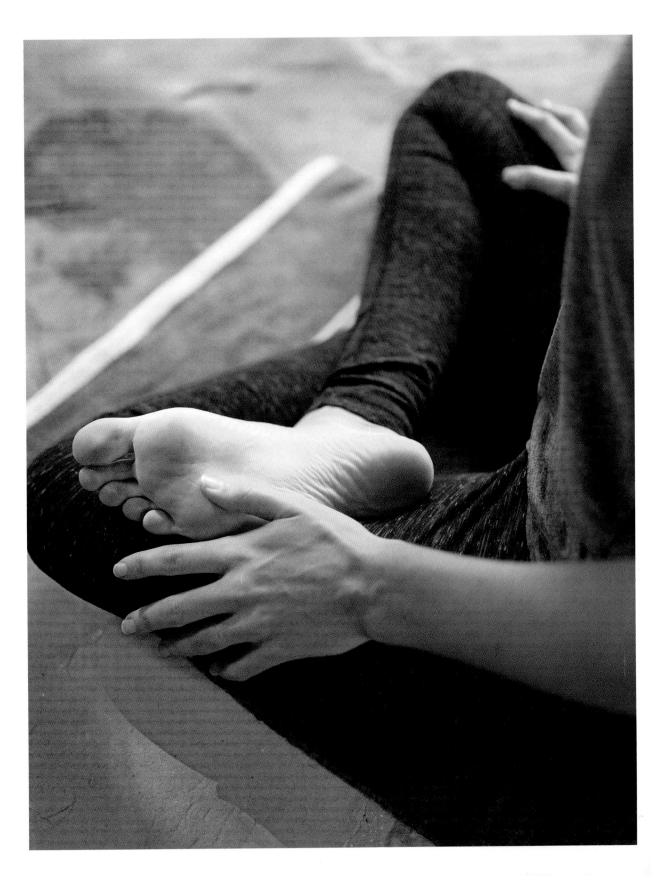

Index

Underscored page references indicate sidebars and tables. **Boldface** references indicate illustrations and photographs.

Batch-cooking, 225, 226, 227

Beans, avoided in elimination phase, 68

Beck, M. N., 149

Bedroom environment, for better sleep, 245, 246, 247, 248

Bedtime, consistent, 249

Bedtime rituals, 110–11, 110

Beef
    Apple-Beet Burgers with Parsnip Fries and Horseradish Spread, **196**, 197
    Balsamic Beef Stew, **184**, 185
    Beef Curry Soup, **192**, 193
    Butternut Breakfast Bake, **176**, 177
    Hidden Liver Chili, **188**, 189
    Nutrivore's Breakfast, 176–77, **177**
    Steak Salad with Spring Veggies, **210**, 211

Beef jerky, 238

Beef liver
    anemia reversed by, 70
    Bacon-Beef Liver Pâté with Rosemary and Thyme, **172**, 173
    Hidden Liver Chili, **188**, 189
    Nutrivore's Breakfast, 176–77, **177**

Beets
    Apple-Beet Burgers with Parsnip Fries and Horseradish Spread, **196**, 197

Bile insufficiency, 90

Biofeedback technician, 32

Biologic DMARDs, 21

Blood disorders, 3

Blood-sugar imbalances
    from chronic stress, 120
    from excess sugar, 57–58
    sleep disturbances and, 98, 104, 104

Blue light, effect on sleep, 94, 106, 126

Blue-light-blocking glasses, 106

Blue-light therapy lamp, 106

Body acceptance, 136

Body-image struggles, 134

Body scan, in bedtime ritual, 110, 111

Bone Broth, 168–69, **169**

Bone strength, exercise for, 132

Book clubs, 156–57

Borbély, Alexander, 95

Bowel movements, tracking, 23

Brain, social pain experienced by, 149, 150

Brain fog, from chronic stress, 120

Breakfasts
    Butternut Breakfast Bake, **176**, 177
    Double Pork Pesto Patties with Wilted Chard, 182, **183**
    in 4-Week Meal Plan, 228–31
    Green Breakfast Soup, 180–81, **181**
    nontraditional, 164
    Nutrivore's Breakfast, 176–77, **177**

Breathe step, xi, xii. *See also stress-related entries*
    in 12-Week Lifestyle Plan, 246–56

Broccoli
    Emerald Salmon with Zesty Green Sauce, 199

Broth
    Bone Broth, 168–69, **169**
    nutrients in, 71

Burgers
    Apple-Beet Burgers with Parsnip Fries and Horseradish Spread, **196**, 197

Burnout, signs of, 118, 120

Butternut squash
    Butternut Breakfast Bake, **176**, 177
    Lemongrass-Scented Chicken Stew, 190–91, **191**

C

Cabbage
    Fermented Vegetables, 174

Caffeine
    reducing intake of, 103
    reliance, from chronic stress, 120
    sleep disturbances from, 98

Cancer
    from autoimmune treatments, 20, 21
    preventing, 132, 160

Carbohydrates
    effect on sleep, 98, 103–4, 104
    elimination-diet-friendly starchy, 91
    insufficient intake of, 90–91
    intolerance to, 89

Cardio obsession, 135

excessive movement and, 134
relationships lowering, 150
in stress response, 115, 116
Counselor, 31
Craft projects, 156
Crohn's disease
in families, 4
integrating therapies for, 35
surgery for, 21, 45
testing for, 18
CRP (C-reactive protein) test, 19
CSA (Community Supported Agriculture), 241
Curry
Beef Curry Soup, **192**, 193
Curried Chicken Salad, **206**, 207
Cycling, 143

journaling about, 23–24

returning in reintroduction phase, 80

treating, 20–22

types of, xi, xii, xiii, 2

variations of, 2, 8

Systemic lupus erythematosus, testing for, 16, 18

T

Tagine

Lamb Tagine with Cauliflower "Rice," 198

Tai chi, 142

Tapioca starch/flour, 237

Tea, caffeine in, 98, 103

Technology, improving relationship with, 126–27, 127

Temperature, for sleep quality, 102

Tests, for self-evaluation. *See* Self-tests and checklists

Tests, medical, 15–16

antibody, 16, 18

determining organ damage and/or inflammation, 18

functional medicine, 19–20

general, related to overall health, 18–19

selectivity about, 48–49

Thyme

Bacon-Beef Liver Pâté with Rosemary and Thyme, **172**, 173

Thyroid antibodies tests, 16

Thyroid panel, 19

Time management, for meal planning, 226–27

TNF inhibitors, 21

Tools, kitchen, 227, 236, 265

Toxic exposures, autoimmune diseases from, 4

Tracking tips, for symptom journal, 23–24

Treadmill desk, 140, 145

Treatments

common medical, 20–21

inadequacy of, 2

medication or surgery, 44–45

natural, 21–22

Treats, 58, 227

Granitas, **218**, 219

Lemon Pie Date Balls, 216, **217**

No-Bake Lemon-Vanilla "Cheesecake," 222–23, **223**

Raspberry Pudding, 220, **221**

Roasted Stone Fruit, **214**, 215

Trevelyan, G.M., 147

Tuna

Tuna Salad with Avo or Garlic "Mayo," 212, **213**

Turmeric

Spatchcocked Chicken with Turmeric Veggies, **202**, 203

12-Week Lifestyle Plan

overview of, 243–44

preparation list for, 257

slow implementation of, 259–60

week 1, 245

week 2, 246

week 3, 247

week 4, 248

week 5, 249

week 6, 250

week 7, 251

week 8, 252

week 9, 253

week 10, 254

week 11, 255

week 12, 256

U

Ulcerative colitis

surgery for, 21, 45

testing for, 18

Ultrasound tests, 18

Underlying conditions, sleep disturbances from, 110

Unexpected major life event, as stressor, 117

Unsupportive relationships, addressing, 153–54, 250

Upper endoscopy, 18

Urgent care clinic, 49